THE ULTIMATE HANDBOOK: HOW TO NAVIGATE THE HORRORS OF OUR HEALTHCARE SYSTEM WITH CONFIDENCE

PROVEN STRATEGIES FOR POSITIVE PATIENT CARE AND HOW TO GET IT

ROBIN SNEAD, M.D.

CONTENTS

Prologue   9
Introduction   11

JUNE'S STORY   17
Ignored by Her Plastic Surgeon   21
June's First Episode of Presyncope and Being Ignored by Her PCP   22
June's Second Presycopal Episode   23
Informing the Hospitalist of the Chest CT Results and Our Conclusion   24
June Scheduled for Discharge Without Further Evaluation   24
Do Not Sign the Discharge Papers   26
This Third Attack Brought June Closer to Death   27
Finally, a Name for Her Condition, But the Physicians Refused to Treat It   27
An Interception from Paris   28
A Hero from Paris Heard Our Pleas, Ordered a Pacemaker, and Saved Her Life   28
The Alarming Rise in Iatrogenic Deaths   29

About the Author: Experience and Perspective   31

1. UNDERSTANDING MANAGED CARE SYSTEMS   33
The Origins of Managed Care: A Historical Perspective   34
Key Legislative Milestones Shaping Managed Care   34
The Structure and Functioning of Managed Care Organizations (MCO)   35
Economic Incentives and Their Impact on Patient Care   37
Ethical Concerns in Managed Care   38
Patient Advocacy in the Managed Care System   38
Conclusion: Navigating Managed Care with Knowledge and Advocacy   39

2. THE PATIENT'S GUIDE TO NAVIGATING MANAGED CARE ... 41
   Mastering the Managed Care Maze: Step-by-Step Navigation ... 42
   Understanding and Utilizing Your Insurance Plan ... 45
   The Role of Primary Care Providers (PCPs) in Managed Care ... 47

3. COMMON PITFALLS AND HOW TO AVOID THEM ... 49
   Long Waiting Times: Strategies for Faster Appointments ... 50
   Prior Authorization Hurdles: How to Expedite Approval ... 51
   Avoiding the Trap of Cost-Cutting Measures ... 53

4. ADVOCATING FOR YOURSELF IN THE HEALTHCARE SYSTEM ... 57
   Understanding the Importance of Healthcare Advocates ... 58
   It Is Very Important to Use Effective Communication with Healthcare Providers ... 60
   Navigating Hospital Discharges: Ensuring Safe Transitions ... 61

5. LEVERAGING TECHNOLOGY FOR BETTER CARE ... 65
   Telehealth: Expanding Access to Care ... 66
   Utilizing Electronic Health Records (EHR) ... 68
   Health Apps and Tools for Managing Your Care ... 70
   Embracing Technology in Your Healthcare Journey ... 72

6. THE POWER OF PREVENTIVE SCREENINGS ... 73
   Benefits of Preventive Screenings ... 74
   The Role of Healthcare Providers ... 77

7. DEALING WITH INSURANCE CHALLENGES ... 79
   You Must Understand Insurance Denials and Appeals ... 80
   Navigating Out-of-Pocket Costs and Copays ... 83
   Choosing the Right Insurance Plan for Your Needs: HMO, PPO, EPO, POS ... 87
   Deductibles and Premiums ... 88
   Open Enrollment: What You Need to Know ... 89

8. CASE STUDIES AND REAL-LIFE SCENARIOS—
INFORMATION PROVIDED TO ME BY NEW OR
ESTABLISHED PATIENTS WHO HAD CONFLICTS
WITH SPECIALISTS 93
   Overcoming Prior Authorization Delays 94
   Reflection Section: Strategies for Overcoming Prior
   Authorization Delays 96
   Effective Self-Advocacy in a Hospital Setting 96
   Managing Chronic Conditions in Managed Care 100
   Ben's Story Is Atypical But Can Be Achieved 103

9. THE IMPACT OF COVID-19 ON MANAGED CARE 107
   COVID-19 and the Exodus of Healthcare Workers 108
   Deaths of Health Care Workers (HCWs) and the End
   of Practicing Medicine 109
   Impact on Patient Care: A Ripple Effect 109
   My Personal Experience as a Patient 110
   COVID-19 Caused Problems for Other Non-
   COVID-19 Patients with Acute and Chronic
   Diseases 111
   Temporary and Traveling Healthcare Workers: The
   Stopgap Solution 112
   Telehealth: Healthcare's New Frontier 112
   Practical Tips for Patients: Navigating Care in a
   Changed World 113

10. ADDRESSING IATROGENIC DEATHS AND
    MEDICAL ERRORS 117
    Understanding Iatrogenic Deaths: A Growing Crisis 118
    Problems of Less Experienced NPs, PAs, and
    Overworked Physicians 119
    The Human and Economic Cost of Medical Errors 120
    Preventing Medical Errors: Strategies for Safer Care 120
    Patient Safety: What You Can Do to Protect Yourself ... 122
    Final Thoughts 123

11. ENHANCING DOCTOR-PATIENT
    RELATIONSHIPS 125
    Building Trust with Your Primary Care Provider 125
    Trust Can Have a Profound Impact on the Doctor-
    Patient Relationship 126
    Reflection Section: Strengthening Your Relationship
    with Your PCP 127

Effective Communication: Asking the Right Questions	128
Reflection Section: Preparing for Your Next Appointment	130
Collaborative Care: Working with Specialists	131
Ending: Summarizing the Main Points	134
12. NAVIGATING HEALTHCARE BUREAUCRACY	**135**
Managing Healthcare Paperwork	136
Settling Disagreements	138
Checklist: Organizing and Managing Healthcare Paperwork	138
Comprehending and Organizing Your Health Records	139
Tips for Managing Health Records	141
Understanding the Referral Process	142
Patient Involvement in the Process	144
Summary of the Referral Process	144
13. ADDRESSING MENTAL HEALTH IN MANAGED CARE	**147**
Meeting Mental Health Needs	148
Overcoming Stigma	149
How to Access Mental Health Services in a Managed Care	150
Navigating Insurance Coverage for Mental Health	151
Alternative Resources for Mental Health Care	151
Integrating Mental and Physical Health Care	153
Strategies for Integrated Care	153
Real-Life Success Story: Janice	154
Conclusion: Whole-Person Health	154
14. LEGAL RIGHTS AND PATIENT ADVOCACY	**155**
The Right to Informed Consent	156
The Right to Access Your Medical Records	157
The Right to Privacy and Confidentiality	157
The Right to Refuse Treatment	158
Reflection Section: Know Your Rights	158
Personal Story	159
Legal Recourse in Cases of Medical Negligence	160
Filing a Medical Malpractice Claim	161

    Utilizing Patient Advocacy Services   161
    Conclusion   163

15. SPECIAL POPULATIONS AND MANAGED CARE   165
    Seniors in Managed Care: Tackling the Challenges   166
    Pediatric Care in the Managed Care System   168
    Managing Chronic Illnesses and Disabilities   170
    Reflection Section: Key Takeaways   173
    Conclusion   173

16. FUTURE TRENDS IN MANAGED CARE   175
    The Future of Telehealth and Digital Health   176
    The Role of Technology in Care Delivery   177
    Innovations in Managed Care Models   179
    Preparing for the Future: Adapting to Change   180
    The Road Ahead   181

    Conclusion   183
    Advocacy Services   189
    Nutrition Tips   193
    Epilogue   199

    References   201
    Author's Bio   207

PROLOGUE

FROM JUNE IN HER OWN WORDS, WITH A SPECIAL MESSAGE AND STORY FOR THE WORLD TO HEAR!

Cancer—a word that sends shivers down the spine and sparks an avalanche of fears and uncertainties. For me, it wasn't just a distant possibility; it became an unwelcome reality three times that has upended my life. However, my journey wasn't just about fighting a disease. It became a testament to the power of advocacy, determination, and courage to confront the illness and the medical challenges that arose along the way.

After my first diagnosis, second diagnosis, and then the third metastatic diagnosis, I entered the labyrinth of treatments, consultations, and endless appointments with a series of doctors. I assumed every doctor would be a guiding light, an expert dedicated to steering me toward recovery. But reality proved to be more complicated. Amid the maze of medical jargon and decisions, I encountered professionals whose carelessness and indifference made me feel like just another name on a chart. The lack of diagnoses, overlooked symptoms, and dismissive attitudes threatened to derail my treatment and jeopardize my chance at survival.

That's when my doctor advocates, Dr. Snead and Dr. Ahmed, stepped in. These heroes refused to let my case slip through the cracks. They spoke often, questioned decisions, demanded second opinions, and held the incompetent accountable. They became my voice when I didn't know what to say or do or was too overwhelmed to speak. These advocates were the difference between life and death for me.

This is the true story of how their unwavering support and expertise became my lifeline. It's a story of resilience in the face of adversity and proof that the right advocates can transform a grim diagnosis into a hopeful battle. It's also a reminder that in the fight against cancer, the people who stand up for you—questioning, challenging, and caring—can make all the difference, especially your doctors. That is what I found in Dr. Snead and Dr. Ahmed. These doctors cared enough to fight for me to have a chance to fight breast cancer three times.

Without them and their relentless and continued advocacy, I would not have a pacemaker, which allowed the doctors to proceed to aggressively provide treatment for this aggressive metastatic cancer that has now taken hold of my body. Having doctors you trust and knowing you are not just another statistic can mean all the difference in the world. Know your doctors and ensure they are the type of doctors who will fight for you to have another chance at living your life!

Thank you, Dr. Snead, for being there to advocate for me. The current world of medicine needs more doctors like you, who are caring, loving, patient, and empathetic, and who advocate for their patients.

INTRODUCTION

It breaks my heart to write about the maleficence I have seen in the healthcare industry. Some of these occurrences are unbelievable; honestly, if I had not witnessed them firsthand, I would not believe them.

Over the last twenty years since the inception of managed care, I have seen the negligence and mistakes made in the name of managed care. Twenty-plus years ago, I started writing about the mishaps of managed care medicine. I wrote about my disgust with how doctors were putting data and believing that keeping track of numbers was more important than putting that effort into good patient care.

THE DEVASTATION OF COVID-19 ON THE HEALTHCARE SYSTEM

However, it has now worsened significantly with the devastation of COVID-19. COVID-19 devastated the world with nightmarish deaths, isolation, and fear. Fear had multiple tentacles that choked and grabbed hold of our mortality, finances, relationships, security, health, hopes, and dreams. For physicians dealing with COVID-19, it shook us to our core. Doctors, along with nurses, were in the trenches. We treated patients with this monster of a disease that, in early 2020, we saw killing people with a horrible, lonely death. Doctors had an unusual group of emotions that included fear of contracting the virus and anxiety about getting answers to defeat this monster.

The ER and intensive care unit doctors faced the most challenges. Except for doctors treating injuries on the battlefield, the ER and ICU docs saw the worst horrific scenes. This disease suffocated their patients, and if they needed to get intubated, it was a rare form of intubation and ventilation that occurred prone, having them lay on their abdomen. The doctors witnessed the patients struggling for their last breath, in an unusually prone position, forced to be isolated and alone.

If that was not horrendous enough, because of the pandemic, these poor patients had to suffer alone without the support, love, or presence of their family or friends. The doctors, along with the nurses, were there bearing witness to their agony, fear, and heart-wrenching loneliness. Depending on their specialty and training, doctors have spent ten to fourteen years preparing to heal, cure, and improve some of the worst medical conditions. But these poor souls were unprepared to partake in the unsurmountable suffering, pain, and fear. They had to put aside these feelings to put in an insane number of hours to treat the never-ending influx of tragically sick COVID-19 patients that were presented.

Doctors often treated these patients with a shortage of PPE (personal protective equipment). I believe this is part of the reason it was found that among doctors aged forty-five to eighty-four, there were 4,511 deaths, 622 more than expected based on pre-pandemic trends in the United States (Kiang et al. 2023). The Centers for Disease Control and Prevention (CDC) reported that, as of April 2021, there were over 400,000 cases of COVID-19 among healthcare personnel in the US, with more than 1,400 deaths. This underscores the significant impact of the pandemic on those in the medical field.

PHYSICIAN SHORTAGE AND THE UNSURMOUNTABLE DEMANDS ON

Managed healthcare and COVID-19 have contributed to the problems we now see in the healthcare system. The issues that I have read about and the ones I have personally seen and have intervened in as a semi-retired physician. I observed a significant increase in the mismanagement of patient care due to the rapid and intrusive rise of managed care in the healthcare system. A POEM (Patient-Oriented Evidence That Matters) article in the *Medical Magazine American Family Physician* this year presented an article outlining an average internal medicine physician with a patient load of 2,000 patients, using guidelines of care and documentation for the top ten chronic illnesses. It would take the average physician 27.3 hours a day to meet the requirements put on them.

Panel size matters. Decreasing the panel size to 1,500 patients decreases the physician's time to sixteen hours daily. Increasing the panel size to 3,000 patients increases the time to 32 hours daily. According to a 2022 report by Definitive Healthcare, Addressing the Healthcare Staffing Shortage, October 2022. Over 117,000 physicians left the profession between the first quarter of 2020 and the last quarter of 2021, followed by 53,000 nurse practitioners, causing a shortage of primary care practitioners, which explains a lot. However, this outflux just increases the burden on the physician who remains practicing. All this contributes to physicians having post-COVID Burnout. These are the reasons: The pressure of managed care medicine demands and the COVID epidemic have caused some of the failures in healthcare that I have witnessed.

The demands of documentation and data keeping associated with a sound Managed Care system and the relentless pain of the COVID-19 pandemic have placed an infallible burden on the Healthcare Industry. Witnessing the results of the fiasco and its harm to patients, I decided to do two things. First, I detailed the gravity of the mistakes made by industry workers. Second, I meticulously detailed patients' strategies to navigate the system in this book.

Over the last fifteen years, I have kept some notes on the errors in the managed care systems that have affected my patients' lives. I did this to write a book that would be fiction based on nonfiction, which I still plan to rewrite in the future. However, I felt compelled to write this book now based on what I have observed in the decline of patient care and the articles I have mentioned regarding the overwork of physicians due to managed care. This unreasonable expectation of doctors and advanced practice providers (NPs and PAs) is one of the reasons, along with burnout from caring for patients during the COVID-19 pandemic, caused a hiatus of over 230,000 healthcare professionals out of the healthcare field. The shortage of healthcare professionals, along with the demands of managed care medicine, is probably one of the reasons, among others, that Iatrogenic deaths have gone up to over 250,000 a year, according to a John Hopkins Study, Makary and Daniel (2016). Other studies state that there are iatrogenic deaths around 400,000 a year.

A CALL TO ACTION

This information, along with the decline I have observed in healthcare over the last thirty-five years and the lack of care my patients have reported receiving in the healthcare system, prompted me to write a book to educate patients on how to navigate the healthcare system to achieve the best possible outcome for themselves.

In this book, I will outline a series of alarming events, one of which nearly cost my dear friend June her life on several occasions. This series of events that almost killed my friend forced me to write this guide to aid patients in navigating the healthcare system to have the best outcomes and to increase healthier longevity.

JUNE'S STORY

June had a series of devastating life-changing encounters with several doctors. June and I have been friends for thirty-five years; we met when I worked at the Doctor's Office Center after completing my internal medicine residency at Rush Presbyterian St. Luke's Hospital. That was my first job as a doctor; I was young, enthusiastic, attentive, and very ambitious. I grew the practice in the first eighteen months from averaging fifteen to sixty-five patients daily, which was not unusual for an acute care center where we saw minor emergencies and performed X-rays and simple surgical procedures.

June was a cheerful young woman who was trained as a teacher but worked as a book salesman at the time. We had similar interests, hit it off, and became good friends. We did what many young, single professional women in Chicago did: We worked hard and played hard.

In the following years, we dated, entertained, and enjoyed living in a culturally dynamic metropolis. I met a handsome, tall, gregarious man, Larry, who became my husband within a year. I was thirty-six, and we decided to have our children quickly. I had two children: my son Akeem, whom I had at age thirty-eight, and my daughter Folasade, whom I had at age forty-one. We called her Sade, after the singer. June became Akeem's godmother, and she is an excellent godmother. She loved dressing Akeem and had a great sense of style in little boys' attire.

Despite being single, June had a strong desire to be a mother. This was possibly because June was not raised by her parents but had a wonderful life raised by her aunt and was part of a large family full of relatives. She decided to adopt a little girl, Kalani, to whom I became a godmother, an honor I shared with another of June's friends. We raised our children with great thought and enthusiasm. Our life of partying and working to maintain a particular lifestyle soon shifted to focusing on the activities that would best promote the happiness and development of our children. We visited amusement parks, hosted elaborate birthday parties, and prioritized their education and after-school activities. We traveled to Walt Disney World in Florida, typically during the Thanksgiving holiday. June was also there for me when I went through a painful, contentious divorce ten years into my marriage. I was June's primary care physician, but at the time, I did not know how important that would be for her.

June developed breast cancer in her fifties. The cancer was an estrogen receptor-positive cancer that was treated with a local lumpectomy and hormonal treatment. June did fine with the treatment; we thought it was gone, not to show its ugly head again. But it did sixteen years later; this time, it was a more aggressive cancer, causing her treatment to be more intense. She had to go in for IV chemotherapy, which usually made her sick with complaints of fatigue, nausea, and vomiting. She did have some problems with not being able to take the first and second choices of chemo that were presented to her because of the adverse side effects. June had an excellent oncologist, Dr. V. A mastectomy was warranted this time around because of the aggressiveness of the cancer. Despite the tumor being located in one breast, June decided to have a double mastectomy, which she believed would decrease her risk of the cancer returning a third time. But before the surgery, she needed to start on chemotherapy after the appropriate testing,

June was referred to a plastic surgeon, Dr. P, by Dr. K, whom we knew and trusted. June went to the plastic surgeon and had a bilateral mastectomy, and Dr. P. prepared June for future bilateral breast implants. I agreed with that decision, even though I did not reveal an opinion. I did not want her to feel pressured. My understanding is that she wanted to feel and appear normal again. Normal means having a female silhouette and feeling attractive in her clothes again. But this was a long, arduous process. Having the breast removed along with the lymph nodes was an invasive, painful surgical procedure.

After healing from the bilateral mastectomy, there was a glimmer of light of normalcy again after the scars healed from the mastectomy. Expanders were planned to be put in to stretch the skin in preparation for the reconstruction and breast implants. Initially, the expanders were tolerable, but they appeared to become larger and form a single, unsightly mass that filled most of her chest wall. June started to complain to the plastic surgeon about pain in her chest wall; he assured her that all women have some pain with the expanders in their chest. After months, he finally decided to evaluate the pain she was having, so he ordered an MRI of her chest.

Mind you, June was under the impression her cancer had gone. She had endured painful chemo infusions, post-chemo nausea, vomiting, and weakness. June had endured the bad taste in her mouth and the loss of her full head of hair. But in all that devastation, she visualized a light at the end of the tunnel. When she felt the overwhelming anxiety, she told herself that this pain and uncertainty were not going to continue forever. The anxiety she felt caused a quickening of her heart and moisture on her brow.

The plastic surgeon sent June for a chest MRI because she complained of chest discomfort. June had a healthy amount of concern but was not fearful of anything horrible creeping up.

June called me that evening, and she sounded distraught. She blurted out, "Did you see my text message?" I said, "No, I've been busy." She said, "Look at it," and abruptly hung up. I believed her anxiety just grabbed hold of me; I went to my text messages and saw she had texted me her online My Chart information, username, password, and website. She wanted me to go to retrieve her MRI report. I used the information to open her chart. I read the report in disbelief; I now understood her unusual behavior on the phone. The only word I saw was metastatic. I quickly felt the urgency to call her to let her know that metastasis does not mean untreatable or a death sentence. And calling June is precisely what I did. At the time, I did not realize the future events that would ensue. Unbeknownst to me, these events made me realize the urgency of telling what I knew about the broken healthcare system.

June was devastated; I heard it in her voice. The first thing I needed to accomplish was to quickly restore her hope. I told her that metastatic disease is not a death sentence; there are new drugs that successfully treat metastatic breast cancer. I told her about my patient who had six different cancers, some diagnosed over twenty-five years ago, and she is fine, with no evidence of cancer. I told her she needed to prepare to get treated again to fight and win the battle with this cancer. The immediate events after her devastating news were hard for me to wrap my head around. June called her oncologist, Dr. A, and the plastic surgeon who ordered the MRI of her chest.

She wanted to know what to do next. Her oncologist, Dr. A, was initially surprised that the MRI revealed metastatic disease in her bone, spine, and liver. Dr. A was very thorough, and all her prior scans and blood tests showed no indication of metastatic disease. But hearing the devastating news, she reassured June and went into fight mode to eradicate this monster.

IGNORED BY HER PLASTIC SURGEON

As for the plastic surgeon, days, weeks, and months had passed, and he had yet to call June to discuss the MRI results he had ordered, despite his office being contacted multiple times by June, who had asked him to call her. She told me he had never called her to discuss her MRI results and any plans or suggestions he might have. June was in disbelief; she had complained for months because of pain in her chest, prompting him to get the MRI finally, and now he was not responding to her calls for some type of plan and or explanation. I was incensed and called and spoke to a female member of his staff. I left a message with her for him to call me and reminded her to inform him that it is malpractice not to respond to June's calls.

As of today, over a year later, neither June nor I have heard from him. Under these circumstances, ignoring June's calls was unusual. I have seen recently that it is not uncommon for patients not to receive a callback, but to ignore the message I left is remarkable.

However, this misstep was only a tiny fraction of the life-threatening problems that June had to navigate, which were to erupt. As bad as this was, it got so much worse. After discovering this devastating news, a list of events occurred in June's life that would shake the strongest individuals to the core.

JUNE'S FIRST EPISODE OF PRESYNCOPE AND BEING IGNORED BY HER PCP

One late afternoon, while I was relaxing and reviewing some charts on my computer, I received a frantic call from my goddaughter, Kalani, stating that her mother, June, had sat down on the toilet and was feeling very dizzy, with difficulty standing up. I spoke to June, and she sounded weak and breathless. She said she felt nauseous and lightheaded and felt like she was going to pass out. I told Kalani to have June lie down and call 911 to get her to the hospital. June had a blood pressure (BP) cuff, and I asked Kalani to give me her BP and pulse readings. Her BP was very low, and her pulse was forty, also low. Usually, when your blood pressure drops, your pulse increases to compensate, but it didn't, which was concerning.

June wanted to get up to use the washroom, but I told Kalani to keep her flat. Standing up with that BP and pulse could cause her to have a stroke. The paramedics finally came; they put in an IV line and gave her normal saline and medicine to increase her pulse. The paramedics took June directly to Hospital X's ER, where she was treated, stabilized, and admitted to the hospital ICU overnight for observation with a cardiac monitor. June was treated for minor electrolyte abnormalities. June was told by the doctors that her BP medication, Coreg, caused her presyncope attack. The medicine Coreg was discontinued, and the nurse told June to follow up with her internist. June's treatment was typical—the episode had abated, and her cardiac workup was normal. Since she was not symptomatic, she was sent home. June was nervous and worried; she had cold shivers when she thought of that whole horrible episode occurring again. She went home and promptly called her current primary care physician at the time. Her doctor did not call back after June left multiple messages. June decided to change primary care physicians.

JUNE'S SECOND PRESYCOPAL EPISODE

A month later, the event occurred again. This time, June felt lightheaded and nauseous. Her blood pressure dropped even lower than the last time, and her pulse was also low again. The pulse was lower than it had been the last time. Again, the paramedics were called, and she was taken to the same hospital as before because when you call an ambulance, they must take you to the nearest hospital. June was seen in the ER. This time, I insisted on speaking to the ER physician and informing him of her history. With that information, the astute ER doctor did a CT scan of her chest.

The CT scan revealed what helped me understand her symptoms. She had a large lymph node near her aortic artery that was probably irritating her vagus nerve; this vagus nerve irritation could explain her low pulse despite her low blood pressure. Typically, when the blood pressure (BP) drops, the pulse increases. I spoke to the ER doctor again, and we agreed that this could cause her low pulse and BP and that she probably needs a pacemaker. June was admitted to the floor; this gave me great relief. Finally, they could do something to stop these attacks. This last one was worse than the first; her pulse was slower, and her BP was barely present. I knew I had to talk to the internist who was caring for her on the floor.

INFORMING THE HOSPITALIST OF THE CHEST CT RESULTS AND OUR CONCLUSION

I called the nursing station, identified myself, and asked the hospitalist, Dr. M, to call me. When the nurses located Dr. M and gave him the message, he did call me. I was anxious to tell him about the discussion I had with the ER doctor about the finding on the CT scan that her symptoms were not primarily due to her heart or her BP dropping. It probably was because of the cancerous LN pressing on her aortic artery, interfering with her vagus nerve, and the significant metastasis surrounding the vascular. I thought she needed to be evaluated for the CT scan results and her need for a pacemaker. Evaluating June solely for a heart abnormality would not be a complete evaluation. Dr. M said he understood the ER doctor had done a CT scan that found a cancerous LN on her aortic artery with metastasis surrounding the vascular tissue. He agreed this might be the etiology of her symptoms and June's need for evaluation for a pacemaker.

JUNE SCHEDULED FOR DISCHARGE WITHOUT FURTHER EVALUATION

June was scheduled to stay in the hospital for further evaluation and treatment. I relaxed and waited to call back after a few hours to see how things were going. To my dismay, when June answered the phone, she informed me that she was being discharged without any further evaluation, except for a heart monitor. This discharge order is when things got crazy. I called the nursing station on the floor and asked them to call the hospitalist I had previously spoken to. The nurse obliged me, and Dr. M called about twenty minutes later. I tentatively asked if he had discharged June, thinking that it was a ridiculous question given our previous conversation about the lymph node on her aorta and the near-death symptoms she was having because of it.

To my surprise, he said yes, that he had discharged her. I asked him why. He said, and I quote, "Because the cardiologist said nothing was wrong with her heart." I then became very annoyed and said we knew her heart was probably not the primary problem causing her to have those near-death attacks. I told the ER doctor's discovery on the CT scan put the etiology of the attacks on the cancerous lymph node pressing on her aortic artery, irritating the vagus nerve. He said he knew. I asked if he had told the cardiologist. He went on to say she had no symptoms while in the hospital! Granted, she was only there for a day. It took everything I could muster not to yell at him. But I calmly said she had a near-death experience twice, probably secondary to the lymph node pressing on her aorta irritating her vagus nerve, which could happen despite her having a normal heart. Then, without addressing my concern, he said she had not had a recurrence in the hospital and had been here long enough.

My voice elevated. I said, "So what? She needs to be evaluated for a pacemaker. She nearly died, and I was on the phone with her daughter and the paramedics when it happened." I asked if he had explained the lymph node to the cardiologist, and he replied that he had. Then, he said she had been here for hours with no recurrence. I screamed at him, stating she needed EP studies and probably a pacemaker. Dr. M still said she must be discharged today. I told him I feared she could die if she went home without further evaluation and treatment because her second attack was worse than her first. I repeated that she should not be discharged without further workup.

He said if she has another attack, she can come back to the ER. I screamed at him and said, "I don't think she can survive another attack!" I asked why they wouldn't perform an EP evaluation to see if a pacemaker was needed. He said, ignoring my question, that she had to be discharged. My daughter was at my home at the time, and she heard me screaming and cursing at this physician. My daughter, who has always been anxious about my health because of my age and the fact her father died after a protracted illness, aggressively told me to calm down.

DO NOT SIGN THE DISCHARGE PAPERS

I called June and told her not to sign the discharge papers. I spoke to the internist again and asked him to transfer her to Hospital Y. He agreed. I called her oncologist, Dr. A, and informed her of the situation. She agreed with me that she needed further evaluation and a pacemaker; the oncologist would then treat the cancerous LN. I asked her if she would accept June for admission at Hospital Y and refer her to a cardiologist, Dr. L, with whom we were familiar. Dr. A agreed; she accepted June for admission and contacted the cardiologist at Hospital Y. June was transferred to Hospital Y that day.

I trusted Dr. L at Hospital Y because I heard from my patients that he was an excellent cardiologist. Dr. A, the oncologist, informed him that the lymph node was pressing on her aorta, as indicated by the chest CT result and her negative cardiac workup. She said she told him of the presyncope episodes June had twice, along with her dangerously low blood pressure and pulse. I relaxed, knowing June was in good hands with two great specialists I trusted. I had retired and was no longer on staff at Hospital Y, so I could not further assist in her care. I spoke to June the following day, and she told me she had already been discharged. Dr. L told June her heart was fine. She was told she did not need a pacemaker. I was disappointed and confused; I still thought she needed a pacemaker. To my dismay, I received another frantic call from her daughter, Kalani, within hours of being discharged from Hospital Y.

THIS THIRD ATTACK BROUGHT JUNE CLOSER TO DEATH

Kalani called me frantic, speaking loud and fast, stating that June passed out cold after going to the toilet and having a bowel movement. This time, she was unconscious. Kalani was unable to obtain a blood pressure reading, and her pulse was slow and weak. She recovered without CPR after the paramedics got there quickly and gave fluids and medication to restore her pulse and BP.

June was transferred to the original Hospital X, where the CT scan revealed the presence of malignant lymph nodes. June was admitted to the hospital after being stabilized in the ER. June got X-rays of her neck, spine, and pelvis. She also had an ECG and blood work. Nothing surprising was revealed; she had a few bony metastases. On the floor, she was placed on a cardiac monitor, which showed an unremarkable rhythm.

FINALLY, A NAME FOR HER CONDITION, BUT THE PHYSICIANS REFUSED TO TREAT IT

A group of cardiologists visited her in the hospital. They tested her heart for abnormalities. However, they did not want to evaluate her for a pacemaker. I asked June to call me when the cardiologist rounded in her room; I wanted to talk to the ones seeing June. I started researching up-to-date medical literature to evaluate June's symptoms of excess vagal nerve stimulation causing her severe loss of pulse and BP. The name of this phenomenon is the Bezold-Jarisch reflex, also known as the vasodepressor reflex.

June handed one of the cardiologists the phone. I told him that I believed she had a vasodepressor reflex. The cardiologist I spoke to said he had never heard of the condition. That frustrated me. In his defense, I later learned that the more common name for the phenomenon was Bezold-Jarisch. I explained to the cardiologist I spoke to that she needed an evaluation for a pacemaker. However, he insisted that she be discharged again. Like before, while she was on the monitor in the hospital, her heart rhythm and BP were normal. I knew if she was discharged again without a pacemaker, she would not survive another attack.

AN INTERCEPTION FROM PARIS

At this time, I became frantic. It was unbelievable not to evaluate June for a pacemaker. Dr. A was ready to treat her cancer more aggressively, but June needed the pacemaker for that to be a possibility. Dr. A and I were on the same page; June needed a pacemaker. We knew a cardiologist on staff at the hospital where June was. I called his office but was told he was on vacation in Paris. I once had his cell phone number, but it was stored in an old tickler file in my office that was packed away and no longer available. But, thank God, Dr. A had his cell number. I told Dr. A about my conversation with the cardiologist. We needed the older, more experienced cardiologist, Dr. K, who knew us and respected our opinion, to instruct the young cardiologists on his team not to discharge June but to have her evaluated for a pacemaker.

A HERO FROM PARIS HEARD OUR PLEAS, ORDERED A PACEMAKER, AND SAVED HER LIFE

From Paris, Dr. K called and had his team cancel her discharge, and he ordered an electrophysiologist to evaluate June, who would assess her for a pacemaker. June received the pacemaker. June was discharged. Her syncopal episodes ceased, and she began to feel better. To no one's surprise, she went back to the hospital for the EP doctor to do a pacemaker check to make sure it was working correctly and also to see if it kicked in and started pacing her heart. Indeed, the pacemaker evaluation revealed that her heart had stopped, and the pacemaker promptly kicked in, possibly saving her life!

THE ALARMING RISE IN IATROGENIC DEATHS

The surge in iatrogenic (induced unintentionally in a patient by a physician) deaths, from an estimated 80,000 in 1990 to nearly 400,000 annually in 2023 (hopkinsmedicine.org), highlights a healthcare system increasingly influenced by cost control over patient care. As patients like June have discovered, the pressure to reduce costs can lead to hasty discharges, limited testing, and reduced treatment options, all of which increase the risk of complications and fatal outcomes. This book aims to help patients understand these risks and navigate the system with greater confidence and advocacy skills.

ABOUT THE AUTHOR: EXPERIENCE AND PERSPECTIVE

With over thirty-five years in medicine, I have seen firsthand the challenges within managed care. My journey as a physician began at Northwestern University's Medical School, now known as the Feinberg School of Medicine, followed by a residency at Rush Presbyterian St. Luke's Hospital. Over the years, I have owned and managed my own practice, as well as multiple healthcare ventures, and co-founded the Independent Practice Association (IPA) Physician Quality Care (PQC) in the 1990s. This experience and several contracts with managed care organizations (MCO) have given me a unique perspective on the realities of the managed care system. I hope to share this knowledge with you.

PURPOSE OF THIS BOOK: A GUIDE TO PATIENT ADVOCACY

This book will equip you with practical tools to navigate the managed care system (MCS), secure necessary care, and advocate effectively for your health. You'll learn strategies for handling prior authorizations, managing long waits, understanding the differences between generic and brand-name drugs, and preparing for doctor's appointments. These are the skills and insights that I have seen are lacking in most patients. I want to help patients navigate these problems, hoping it will empower them to take control of their healthcare to get their desired outcomes.

A CALL TO ACTION

Let us embark on this journey together to explore the realities of the managed care system (MCS). With knowledge, persistence, and advocacy, you can navigate this system effectively, utilizing the necessary tools to protect your health and ensure you receive the quality care you deserve.

CLOSING NOTE

June's story highlights the pressing need for patient advocacy in a healthcare system that frequently prioritizes cost over care. In the following chapters, you will learn how to advocate for yourself or a loved one so you don't have to face the challenges alone. This book is your guide to navigating managed care, and I hope it will empower you to achieve the best possible outcomes in your healthcare journey.

1

UNDERSTANDING MANAGED CARE SYSTEMS

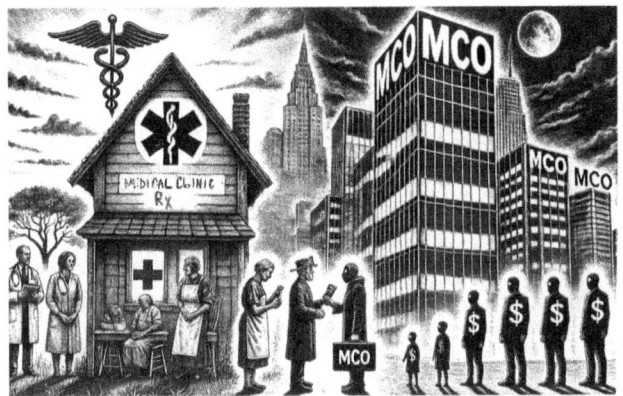

One winter morning, when I had an office full of patients, I received a frantic call from a young mother named Lisa, who had been diagnosed with a rare autoimmune disorder. Lisa's condition had been manageable until her insurance switched to a managed care plan. Suddenly, every aspect of Lisa's treatment was scrutinized. The medication that had kept her symptoms in check was deemed "too expensive," and her referrals to specialists were delayed. Lisa's health slowly deteriorated, illustrating the challenges patients face in the managed care system (MCS). Lisa's experience is not unique, and it reinforced the urgency for me to inform people of the need to understand how these systems operate and how patients can navigate them effectively.

THE ORIGINS OF MANAGED CARE: A HISTORICAL PERSPECTIVE

Managed care systems emerged in the 1970s to control rising healthcare costs and address perceived inefficiencies. Dr. Paul Ellwood, often referred to as the "father of the HMO," pioneered Health Maintenance Organizations (HMOs) to deliver cost-effective care through a network of healthcare providers. This idea gained support with the passage of the Health Maintenance Organization Act of 1973, signed into law by President Nixon, which incentivized the creation of HMOs through federal grants and loans.

By the 1980s, HMOs had become increasingly popular. They focused on preventive care and a strict referral and prior authorization system to avoid the higher costs of hospital treatments. As HMOs surged in popularity, Preferred Provider Organizations (PPOs) emerged. These organizations offered more flexibility by allowing patients to see both in-network and out-of-network providers, though at a higher cost for the latter. PPOs appealed to those seeking more choices without the stringent requirements of HMOs.

KEY LEGISLATIVE MILESTONES SHAPING MANAGED CARE

- **Employee Retirement Income Security Act (ERISA) of 1974**: ERISA preempted state laws that regulated employee

health plans, allowing HMOs and other managed care plans to expand under federal guidelines.
- **Balanced Budget Act of 1997**: This act introduced the Medicare+Choice program (now known as Medicare Advantage), which enabled Medicare beneficiaries to enroll in managed care plans with a focus on controlling Medicare spending.
- **Affordable Care Act (ACA) of 2010**: Promoted Accountable Care Organizations (ACOs), emphasizing coordinated, value-based care and encouraging providers to focus on patient outcomes rather than service volume.

The transition from fee-for-service to managed care was transformative. The traditional fee-for-service model reimbursed providers per service, creating incentives for providers to perform additional procedures. In contrast, managed care introduced capitation models, where providers receive a set amount per patient, incentivizing cost-effective care. However, this shift also led to concerns about undertreatment, as providers could limit procedures to stay within budget.

Understanding this history helps explain the current challenges of the MCS, which often puts cost-saving above patient-centered care.

THE STRUCTURE AND FUNCTIONING OF MANAGED CARE ORGANIZATIONS (MCO)

Managed care organizations (MCOs) come in several forms, each with distinct features. Here's an overview of the four main types:

1. **Health Maintenance Organizations (HMOs):** Require members to choose a primary care physician (PCP) as a

gatekeeper for all services, including specialist referrals. While HMOs emphasize cost savings and preventive care, they restrict patients to in-network providers, often requiring prior authorization for specialized care. Failure to obtain referrals or seek care outside the network typically results in no coverage.
2. **Preferred Provider Organizations (PPOs):** Offer flexibility, allowing members to see both in-network and out-of-network providers (at a higher cost). No referrals are required, making PPOs attractive to those seeking choice and willing to pay more.
3. **Exclusive Provider Organizations (EPOs):** A middle ground between HMOs and PPOs, EPOs require members to use in-network providers but do not mandate referrals for specialists, balancing cost and accessibility.
4. **Point-of-Service (POS) Plans:** Point-of-service (POS) plans combine elements of HMO and PPO plans. Members must choose a PCP and need specialist referrals, but they can see out-of-network providers at a higher cost. POS plans offer structure with flexibility.

The Internal Workings of MCOs

- **Provider Networks and Credentialing:** MCOs create networks of providers who meet specific quality and cost standards. Credentialing verifies that providers are qualified and capable of delivering high-quality care.
- **Utilization Management and Review:** Patients should be aware that Managed Care Organizations (MCOs) utilize prior authorizations and reviews to evaluate the necessity and effectiveness of treatments, aiming to prevent costly or unnecessary procedures.

- **Care Coordination and Case Management:** MCOs employ coordinators and case managers to assist patients with complex needs, ensuring comprehensive care and reducing hospital readmissions. In my opinion, these services are underutilized.
- **Quality Assurance and Performance Monitoring:** MCOs track provider performance, patient satisfaction, and health outcomes using metrics such as Health Effectiveness Data and Information Set (HEDIS), continuously improving standards of care.

ECONOMIC INCENTIVES AND THEIR IMPACT ON PATIENT CARE

Economic incentives within the MCS heavily influence medical decision-making, often pressuring providers with more significant monetary bonuses to adopt cost-saving measures, like using generic medications or limiting hospital stays. These strategies, while reducing costs, can sometimes compromise patient outcomes. I remember one of the MCSs I was involved in coming to my office every month to talk about cost-saving measures, my particular metrics, and occasionally my bonuses.

Impact of Economic Incentives on Treatment Quality

- **Under-treatment:** Economic constraints may lead providers to avoid necessary treatments to stay within budget, potentially compromising patient care. I have ex-patients complain to me of considerable gaps in the treatment they have received, not just from economic restraints. However, from the physician's perspective, they are frustrated, overworked, and underpaid, leading to

activities that are not driven by financial constraints, such as not conducting complete physical exams, decreasing callbacks, and allowing patients to interpret their own results on electronic health records.
- **Over-Treatment:** The fee-for-service model incentivizes the provision of more services, thereby increasing overall costs and the risk of unnecessary procedures.
- **Capitation and Value-Based Models:** Capitation models incentivize preventive care but may lead to undertreatment. In contrast, value-based models link reimbursement to patient outcomes, cultivating provider collaboration to improve care.

ETHICAL CONCERNS IN MANAGED CARE

I occasionally felt uneasy when the MCA staff came to my office to discuss cost savings, my specific statistics, and what I could do to improve them. Managed care often presents moral dilemmas as providers weigh cost control against quality care. Financial incentives should never compromise patient health, yet systemic pressures can disproportionately impact patients from lower socioeconomic backgrounds, leading to disparities in care access.

PATIENT ADVOCACY IN THE MANAGED CARE SYSTEM

Patients can proactively navigate the MCS by:

- **Asking About Treatment Options:** Patients must inquire about the effectiveness and costs of recommended treatments to make informed decisions.
- **Understanding Coverage:** Familiarize yourself with what your plan covers and what requires prior authorization.

- **Appealing Denials:** If you are denied necessary treatment, gather documentation from your provider and submit a formal appeal. Persistence and well-documented appeals can lead to successful outcomes.

For example, a patient needing a costly medication may initially be denied insurance coverage. However, they can often reverse the decision by submitting medical evidence and a well-documented appeal. Engaging a patient advocate can also help them navigate these complexities.

Proactive Tips for Patients

- **Be Informed**: Understanding the structure of your MCO and its coverage can help prevent unexpected surprises.
- **Prepare for Appointments**: Bring questions about alternative treatments, side effects, and costs.
- **Request a Second Opinion**: If a treatment feels insufficient, seeking another opinion can ensure you're receiving appropriate care.

CONCLUSION: NAVIGATING MANAGED CARE WITH KNOWLEDGE AND ADVOCACY

The managed care system shapes the experiences of patients and providers alike, often emphasizing cost control over comprehensive care. By understanding the historical context, structure, and economic incentives within managed care, patients can more effectively navigate the system and advocate for their own health. The following chapters will build on this foundation, providing specific strategies for managing prior authorizations, addressing delays, and securing necessary treatments.

Empowered with knowledge, patients can take control of their healthcare journey and ensure they receive quality care in a system that may not always prioritize it.

2

THE PATIENT'S GUIDE TO NAVIGATING MANAGED CARE

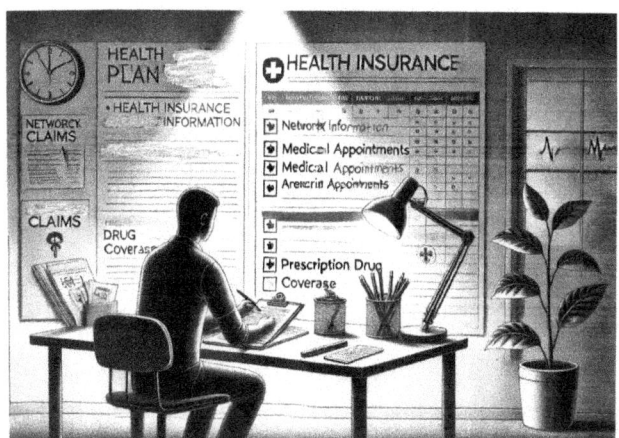

On a busy summer afternoon in my office, I met a new patient, Rachel, a mother who had spent six exhausting months entangled in the managed care system (MCS) for her son's rare neurological condition. She shared her frustration over repeated referrals, denials, and endless paperwork. Rachel's experience highlights the importance of a clear, step-by-step roadmap for navigating MCS. I provide just that in this chapter, offering actionable steps for effectively managing your care within this system.

MASTERING THE MANAGED CARE MAZE: STEP-BY-STEP NAVIGATION

Navigating an MCS starts with selecting the right insurance plan and understanding its structure.

Initial Enrollment: Choosing the Right Plan

- **Evaluate Your Needs:** Assess your health history and anticipated yearly needs.
- **Compare Plans:** Review benefits, premiums, deductibles, and provider networks. Doing this can save you money.
- **Check Medication Coverage:** Ensure essential medications are on the formulary (list of covered drugs).
- **Utilize Open Enrollment:** This annual period allows you to adjust your plan based on changes in your health or financial situation.

Selecting Providers and Staying In-Network

- **Choose a primary care physician (PCP)**: Your PCP will coordinate your care, so choose one based on credentials, experience, and patient reviews.
- **Stay In-Network**: Using in-network providers typically results in lower out-of-pocket costs. Your PCP can refer you to specialists in the network when needed.

Scheduling Preventive Services and Check-Ups

- **Routine Screenings and Vaccinations**: Many preventive services are fully covered, saving you money.
- **Annual Check-Ups**: Regular visits help detect issues early and maintain overall health. Skipping these is a mistake.

Preparing for Appointments

- **List Questions and Concerns**: Write down any issues you want to discuss.
- **Bring Medical Records**: Include past test results and a list of medications to provide your doctor with a comprehensive picture.
- **Understand the Purpose of Your Visit**: Whether a routine check-up or follow-up, being clear on the appointment's focus ensures you get the most out of the time.

Keeping Organized Health Records

- **Utilize Digital Tools:** Patient portals and apps facilitate easier access to your medical records, test results, and appointment schedules.
- **Health Journal**: Track symptoms, treatments, and side effects in a personal health journal to monitor your progress and facilitate adjustments in your care.

Managing Common Obstacles

- **Denied Claims**: Review the denial letters to understand the reasons for the denials. Follow up with your provider and insurance company and, if necessary, go through the appeals process. This typically involves providing

additional information to strengthen your case. Your PCP can help you with this.
- **Referral Process**: Ensure your PCP's office forwards referrals for testing to specialists and that all parties, including the specialist's office, confirm receipt. In my experience, referrals are not one of the most favored tasks for doctors to undertake. So you need to stay on top of this.
- **Prescription Drug Coverage**: If a prescribed medication isn't covered, ask about alternatives or request a formulary exception. Newer medications often have fewer side effects and are more effective but more costly. You can discuss this with your PCP.

Quick Checklist for Navigating Managed Care

- **Enrollment**:
    - Review your needs, compare plans, and check medication coverage.
- **Provider Selection**:
    - Choose a qualified PCP within your network; you typically pay more if they are out of network.
- **Appointment Prep**:
    - You should bring questions about your medical records, stay focused on the visit's goals, and ensure you bring notes on topics you must cover. You can't afford to be unprepared. These appointments may be short, and the doctor may be very busy. Your goal is to get as much care out of this visit as possible.
- **Health Records**:
    - Utilize digital tools and maintain a health journal.

- **Overcoming Obstacles**:
  - Denied claims, managed referrals, and checked prescription coverage.

UNDERSTANDING AND UTILIZING YOUR INSURANCE PLAN

Essential Components of Insurance Plans You Need to Know

- **Premiums**: The monthly amount you pay to keep your insurance active
- **Deductibles**: The amount you pay out-of-pocket before insurance kicks in
- **Copayments**: A set service fee, like $30 for a doctor's visit
- **Coinsurance**: A percentage of costs you pay after meeting your deductible (e.g., 20 percent)

In-Network vs. Out-of-Network Services

- **In-Network Providers**: Offer discounted rates with lower out-of-pocket costs
- **Out-of-Network Providers**: Often result in higher charges, so confirm your provider's network status before scheduling appointments

Using the Explanation of Benefits (EOB)

- Your insurance sends an EOB aftercare outlining the billed amount, insurance coverage, and your responsibility. This summary clarifies any financial obligations but is not a bill.

Choosing the Right Plan During Open Enrollment

- **Compare Plan Types**: HMO, PPO, EPO, and POS plans vary in flexibility and cost.
- **Assess Health Needs**: If you need regular care, a plan with a higher premium but lower out-of-pocket costs may be more economical.

Maximizing Your Insurance Benefits

- **Preventive Care and Wellness Programs**: Take advantage of free screenings, vaccinations, and wellness visits to avoid costly treatments later.
- **Telehealth**: Often less expensive and more convenient for consultations.
- **Health Savings Accounts (HSAs) and Flexible Spending Accounts (FSAs)**: These accounts allow you to set aside pre-tax dollars for medical expenses, reducing your taxable income.

Managing Disputes and Claims

- **File and Track Claims**: Keep copies of documentation and monitor your claim's status.
- **Handling Denials**: Common reasons include claim errors or "not medically necessary" labels. Effective appeals often involve a detailed letter and supporting documents.
- **Seek Help from State Resources**: State insurance commissions can mediate disputes if needed.

THE ROLE OF PRIMARY CARE PROVIDERS (PCPS) IN MANAGED CARE

The Vital Role of Your PCP

- **Routine Check-Ups and Preventive Screenings**: Regular visits allow PCPs to monitor and catch potential health issues early.
- **Coordinating Specialty Care**: When necessary, your PCP arranges specialist care and ensures they have relevant medical records for seamless care.

Choosing a PCP Wisely

- **Credentials and Experience**: Look for board-certified providers with experience in conditions similar to yours.
- **Communication Style**: Choose a PCP who listens, explains clearly, and makes you comfortable.

Accessibility and Convenience

- **Location and Office Hours**: Choose a conveniently located PCP with hours that suit your schedule. Check for online booking or telehealth options.

Building a Strong Relationship with Your PCP

- **Communicate openly**: Share your health goals and concerns so your primary care physician (PCP) can tailor their advice to your specific needs.
- **Participate in Shared Decision-Making**: Collaborate on treatment choices for more tailored care.

- **Follow-Up on Tests and Referrals**: Always check for test results and referral progress to ensure continuity of care.

Practical Steps for Working with Your PCP

- **Prepare for Visits**:
    - List symptoms and questions.
    - Be open and thorough with information.
- **Discuss Treatment Options**:
    - Raise concerns about specific treatments; your PCP may suggest alternatives.
- **Stay Updated**:
    - Don't assume no news is good; follow up on results and next steps.

By following these steps, patients can better navigate the managed care system and build strong relationships with providers, ensuring they receive the highest quality of care. This chapter emphasizes clarity, simplicity, and actionable guidance, helping patients like Rachel navigate managed care confidently and effectively.

3

COMMON PITFALLS AND HOW TO AVOID THEM

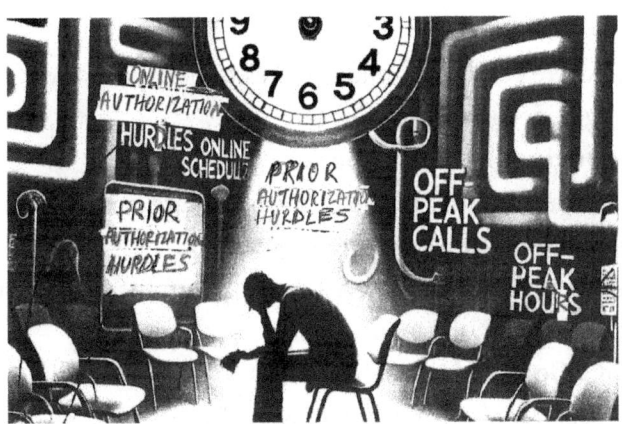

Navigating the managed care system (MCS) can often feel like solving an intricate puzzle. I had a patient, Patricia, who was a busy mother and came in complaining of anxiety because she spent weeks trying to secure an appointment for her daughter's persistent pain. She encountered common pitfalls that led to her frustration and anxiety because of the delays and compromised care her daughter was getting. This chapter covers practical strategies for addressing three common challenges: long waiting times, prior authorization hurdles, and cost-cutting measures.

LONG WAITING TIMES: STRATEGIES FOR FASTER APPOINTMENTS

Securing timely appointments is a common challenge; tackling it requires more than simply calling your doctor's office. Here are strategies to improve your chances of getting the care you need quickly:

- **Use Online Booking Systems and Patient Portals**
    - Book appointments at your convenience.
    - Access real-time slot availability to choose what works best for you.
    - Receive reminders and updates to help you stay organized.
- **Call During Off-Peak Hours**
    - Try calling early in the morning or late in the afternoon when hold times may be shorter.
    - Request to be placed on a cancellation list, which can open up appointments sooner.
- **Build a Good Relationship with Office Staff**
    - Regularly check for any new openings.
    - Express appreciation for their help; they may be more likely to notify you if a spot becomes available.
- **Consider Alternative Options for Immediate Care**
    - Urgent care centers offer timely care for non-emergency issues with shorter waits.
    - Telehealth services enable you to consult a healthcare provider from home for follow-up or minor issues.
    - Nurse hotlines provide immediate advice, often available through your insurance.

- **Plan Ahead and Book Next Appointments Early**
  - Schedule follow-ups before leaving your current appointment to ensure continuity.
  - Keep a calendar for upcoming medical needs, routine check-ups, and reminders.

Checklist for Reducing Wait Times

- **Utilize online tools, such as patient** portals and appointment reminders.
- **Strategic Calling Times**: Call during less busy hours and request cancellation list placement.
- **Proactive Communication**: Build rapport with office staff and regularly check availability.
- **Alternative Care Options**: Urgent care, telehealth, and nurse hotlines are helpful.
- **Plan Ahead**: Schedule follow-ups promptly and track appointments effectively.

Implementing these strategies can help you reduce the frustration of long waiting times, enabling timely access to medical care.

PRIOR AUTHORIZATION HURDLES: HOW TO EXPEDITE APPROVAL

Prior authorization—insurance company approval before receiving specific treatments or medications—can often feel like a bureaucratic maze. It involves submitting documentation about the treatment's necessity and sometimes facing delays or denials.

Here's how to navigate and speed up this process:

- **Ensure Complete and Accurate Documentation**
    - Have your healthcare provider submit all necessary details, including diagnosis, history, and rationale for treatment.
- **Follow Up Regularly**
    - Contact your insurance company to verify the status and inquire if any additional information is required. Persistence can speed up your request.
- **Involve Your Healthcare Provider**
    - Request that your doctor follow up with the insurance company, as their input can influence approval. Remember the saying, "The squeaky wheel gets the oil."
- **Use Patient Advocacy Services**
    - Patient advocates are skilled in dealing with insurance companies, helping gather documentation, and communicating with your insurer on your behalf.
    - I include a list of advocacy programs in the last chapters of this book.
- **Prepare for Denials and Appeal if Necessary**
    - If denied, review the denial letter to understand the reason, then gather additional documentation.
    - Write a clear appeal letter that addresses the reasons for the denial, supported by relevant medical records and input from the provider.
    - If needed, contact your state's insurance commission for additional support.
- **Plan Ahead**
    - Start the authorization process early for any treatment you anticipate needing. This proactive approach helps ensure approvals are in place before you need care.

Checklist for Expediting Prior Authorization

- **Complete Documentation**: Submit all required information upfront.
- **Regular Follow-Ups**: Stay persistent with status checks.
- **Provider Involvement**: Request follow-ups with the doctor's insurance (very important).
- **Patient Advocacy Services**: Engage advocates to assist in appeals.
- **Prepare for Appeals**: Understand the reasons for denial and gather extra documentation.
- **Plan Ahead**: Start the authorization process in advance.

Following these steps can streamline prior authorization, helping you get the necessary treatments and medications on time.

AVOIDING THE TRAP OF COST-CUTTING MEASURES

Cost-cutting measures, such as prescribing generics or shortening hospital stays, are standard in managed care but can affect patient outcomes. Here's how to navigate and advocate for the care you need:

- **Discuss Alternatives and Advocate for Your Needs**
    - If a generic doesn't work for you, request the brand-name version. Ask your provider to document the medical necessity, as this can help ensure insurance coverage approval.
- **Seek a Second Opinion for Complex Conditions**
    - For more complicated cases, getting another specialist's input can confirm treatment needs and support requests for insurance approval.

- **Communicate Effectively with Your Provider**
    - Be open about any concerns or reservations you may have regarding treatments. Your provider can document these in your records, reinforcing your need for specific care.
- **Stay Informed and Research Options**
    - Knowing your coverage, prior authorization requirements, and out-of-pocket costs can help you prepare for and navigate cost-cutting limitations. Familiarity with options can aid in deciding the best treatment path.
- **Utilize Patient Support Groups and Online Resources**
    - These resources offer shared experiences and strategies from others who have navigated similar situations. They can also provide updated information and tools for advocating effectively within the MCS.

Checklist for Avoiding Cost-Cutting Pitfalls

- **Alternative Options:** Discuss brand-name options if generics are ineffective.
- **Second Opinion**: Seek additional input for complex cases.
- **Clear Communication**: Be upfront with providers about your needs.
- **Stay Informed**: Research treatment options and insurance policies.
- **Patient Resources**: Leverage support groups and online tools.
- **Speak Up:** Don't be intimidated into silence; speak up for yourself!

You can advocate for the care you need despite managed care's financial constraints by communicating openly with providers, seeking second opinions, and staying informed.

By anticipating these common pitfalls and employing practical strategies, you can navigate the complexities of managed care more effectively. Proactive communication, thorough documentation, and informed decision-making can empower you to advocate for the quality healthcare you deserve.

4

ADVOCATING FOR YOURSELF IN THE HEALTHCARE SYSTEM

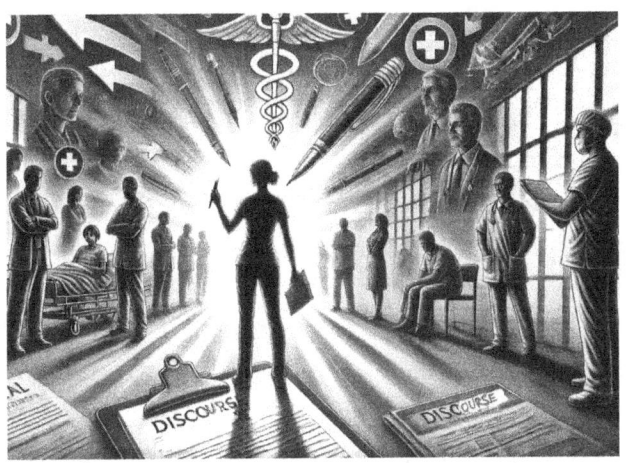

Karen, a patient who had been seeking a diagnosis for months, shared her story on a cold winter's day when I was extremely busy seeing patients with colds and the flu. Karen had been my patient for years, starting as a teenager. She had moved to the East Coast for a job several years prior. She dropped by the office during a visit to Illinois. Karen told me she developed a series of complex neurological symptoms. Karen's illness had her visiting multiple specialists and receiving conflicting information that left her feeling more lost and frustrated.

Instead of giving up, Karen chose to take control of her healthcare journey. She researched her symptoms, documented her health history, and educated herself on her rights as a patient. She did her research and found an excellent, responsive neurologist. Her journey from confusion to empowerment highlights the power and necessity of self-advocacy in today's healthcare system.

UNDERSTANDING THE IMPORTANCE OF HEALTHCARE ADVOCATES

- **Educate Yourself**:
    - Explore reliable medical sources such as the Mayo Clinic, WebMD, and the National Institutes of Health (NIH). Understanding your health condition, treatments, and medical terminology can help you communicate clearly with your providers and make informed decisions.
- **Consider a Healthcare Advocate**:
    - An advocate is important and can be a family member, friend, or professional who supports you during medical appointments, asks important questions, and keeps track of your treatment plan. Advocates are beneficial during times of stress or when facing complex health issues.
- **Build Your Health History File**:
    - Gather past medical records, test results, and information on medications and allergies.
    - Document a timeline of significant diagnoses, treatments, and surgeries to provide a clear health overview.

- Having this information ready aids you and your healthcare providers in delivering informed, consistent care.
- **Know Your Rights as a Patient**:
  - "Informed consent" means understanding and consenting to any treatment while being fully aware of its risks, benefits, and alternatives.
- **Access to Medical Records**:
  - Under HIPAA, you can access your medical records anytime.
- **Second Opinions**:
  - If you are unsure about a diagnosis or treatment, you can seek a second opinion from another healthcare provider.
- **Patient Advocacy Resources**:
  - The Patient Advocate Foundation (PAF) offers case management, financial aid, and educational resources.
  - Hospital patient advocates can help resolve issues within the hospital, like billing disputes or communication challenges.
  - Online support communities such as PatientsLikeMe or HealthUnlocked provide large online platforms for sharing experiences, seeking advice, and connecting with others facing similar issues.

Reflection: Your Personalized Health History

Take some time to collect your medical records and medication information, and document your health history. By organizing this information, you will be better prepared for medical appointments and a more effective advocate for your care.

IT IS VERY IMPORTANT TO USE EFFECTIVE COMMUNICATION WITH HEALTHCARE PROVIDERS

Of all the information I have listed in this book, the following five points are important for receiving the best health care in the Managed Care System.

- **Prepare for Appointments:**
    - List your symptoms and any questions ahead of time to make the most of your time with the provider. Many of my patients fail to do this.
    - Bring a friend or family member for support who can help remember details and provide emotional support. This helps you, and I find it makes it easier for the doctor to understand the gravity of the situation.
    - Take notes during your visit to capture essential instructions and follow-up steps.
- **Describe Symptoms Clearly**:
    - Use specific terms to communicate effectively with your doctor. I suggest avoiding vague language; for example, instead of saying, "I feel off," describe precise symptoms like "I've had a sharp pain in my upper abdomen for five days, especially after meals."
- **Clarify and Summarize**:
    - Don't be afraid to ask for clarification on medical terms or instructions you don't understand.
    - Summarize the provider's instructions and repeat it to them in your own words to ensure you understand the treatment plan.
- **Practice Assertiveness**:
    - Don't hesitate to inquire about all available treatment options and ask for written follow-up instructions.

- If a treatment plan doesn't align with your preferences or goals, voice your concerns. Your healthcare provider should be willing to discuss alternative options.
- Be on top of and inquire and be assertive about any prior authorizations that are pending.
- **Build a Collaborative Relationship:**
  - Share your health goals and preferences with your provider to tailor the care plan to your needs.
  - If you cannot adhere to a prescribed regimen, be honest about it—your doctor may be able to adjust the plan.
  - Don't hesitate to provide feedback on your treatments to ensure your care remains effective and supportive. I have always enjoyed working with patients who are actively involved in their own healthcare.

NAVIGATING HOSPITAL DISCHARGES: ENSURING SAFE TRANSITIONS

- **Understand the Discharge Summary:**
  - This document outlines your hospitalization details, treatments, and follow-up care requirements. It's essential to keep this on hand for your primary care physician (PCP) and any future healthcare appointments.
- **Post-Discharge Instructions:**
  - Ensure they are clearly written and informative and that you understand what is being said. I have seen poorly written discharge summaries and instructions. Do not hesitate to ask for clarification on anything you do not understand.

- Review your medication schedule, wound care instructions, activity restrictions, and dietary guidelines before leaving.
- Learn about any warning signs, such as fever or increased pain, that would signal a need for immediate medical attention.

- **Ask Questions Before Leaving:**
  - Clarify any changes in medication, follow-up appointments, and activity or dietary restrictions.
  - Understand when and where follow-up visits and tests should occur and how to proceed with your recovery.
- **Schedule a Post-Discharge PCP Appointment:**
  - This appointment is essential for reviewing your discharge summary and ensuring a smooth transition from hospital to home. It allows your PCP to monitor your recovery and make necessary adjustments to your care plan. Unfortunately, this is ignored if a patient is feeling better. Do not make this mistake.
- **Utilize Community Resources**:
  - Home Health services provide in-home care, such as medication management and physical therapy, to support recovery.
- **Support Groups:**
  - Local and online support groups can offer practical advice, emotional support, and community connection during recovery. Online support communities such as PatientsLikeMe, HealthUnlocked, and others can be helpful.

Checklist: Key Questions Before Leaving the Hospital

Don't be afraid to speak up and get the necessary medical care.

- **Medication Changes and Instructions**:
    - What new medications am I being prescribed?
    - When and how should I take these medications?
    - Are there any potential side effects to monitor?
- **Follow-up appointments and Tests**:
    - Ask the hospitalist about any follow-up appointments that are needed and where they will be held.
    - Do I need to arrange any additional tests?
    - Who should I contact if I need to change an appointment?
- **Activity and Dietary Restrictions That Need to Be Sorted Out**:
    - Are there specific activities I should avoid?
    - Do I need to make dietary changes?
    - How long do these restrictions apply?

Understanding the discharge process and asking essential questions before leaving the hospital ensures a smoother recovery journey. Effective communication with your PCP and leveraging available community resources will help you confidently navigate this transition.

Self-advocacy within the managed care system is essential for receiving the care you deserve. Educating yourself, preparing thoroughly for appointments, establishing clear communication with providers, and utilizing resources can empower you to navigate healthcare challenges successfully and ensure a more satisfying experience.

5

LEVERAGING TECHNOLOGY FOR BETTER CARE

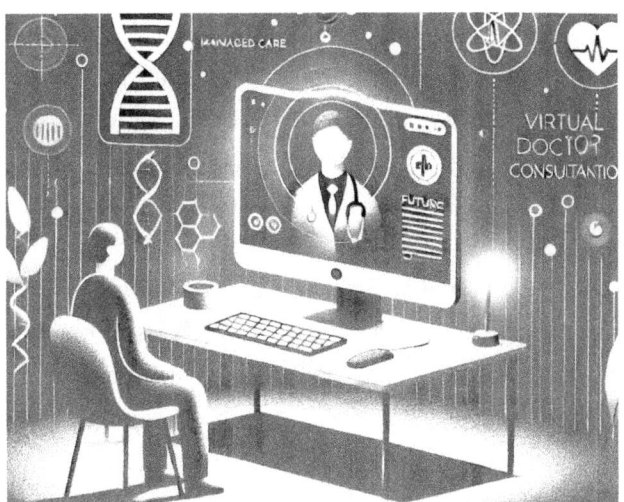

A previous patient, John, an elderly man who moved to a remote town, shared his struggle with managing his uncontrolled diabetes due to limited access to specialized care. Regular visits were nearly impossible, with the closest dietitian over 100 miles away. John's health journey changed when he was introduced to telehealth, which allowed him to consult with a dietitian virtually, improving his condition management from the comfort of his home. His story illustrates the transformative power of technology in expanding access to healthcare.

TELEHEALTH: EXPANDING ACCESS TO CARE

I personally love telehealth, and I started to use it in my practice during the pandemic. It has revolutionized healthcare delivery, particularly for those in remote or underserved areas. Key benefits include:

- **Convenience of Virtual Consultations**: There is no travel involved and no lengthy wait times. You can consult with healthcare providers from home, saving time and reducing stress.
- **Reduced Travel Time and Costs**: Telehealth eliminates long journeys and associated expenses, which is particularly beneficial for those in rural areas.
- **Increased Access to Specialists:** Connect with specialists from afar, avoiding delays in diagnoses and treatment plans.
- **Continuity of Care in Emergencies**: During COVID-19, telehealth minimized virus transmission risks, enabling ongoing care without physical visits. I personally was grateful because of my age and the increased risk of a bad outcome with COVID-19.

Types of Telehealth Services

1. **Video Consultations**: Discuss symptoms, receive advice, and get prescriptions without an in-person visit.
2. **Remote Monitoring**: Devices track vitals like blood pressure and glucose, sending real-time data to healthcare

providers. Many of my patients obtained blood pressure and pulse monitors along with the required glucose monitors diabetics obtained.
3. **Teletherapy for Mental Health**: Access mental health support virtually, removing logistical and stigma barriers.
4. **Mobile Health Units and Teletriage**: Mobile units deliver care to underserved areas, while telehealth provides immediate guidance on care needs.

Preparing for a Telehealth Appointment

- **Check Technology**: Have a stable internet connection, a working camera, and a microphone.
- **List Symptoms and Questions**: Write down any symptoms, questions, or changes in your health. These visits typically are shorter than office visits, and preparation is important.
- **Create a Quiet Space**: Choose a private, distraction-free area to ensure a focused and confidential conversation.

Addressing Telehealth Challenges

- **Technical Issues**: Keep troubleshooting tips on hand, like restarting devices or switching to a wired internet connection.
- **Limitations in Physical Exams:** Telehealth can be an initial step, with in-person visits scheduled as needed.
- **Privacy and Security**: Use HIPAA-compliant platforms and discuss privacy policies with providers to protect health information.
- **Insurance Coverage**: Verify coverage of telehealth services with your provider to prevent unexpected costs.

Reflection: Preparing for Your Telehealth Appointment

Ensure your device and internet are ready, and familiarize yourself with the telehealth platform. Prepare a list of symptoms, questions, and concerns, and choose a quiet, private space. These steps help maximize the benefits of your virtual consultation.

UTILIZING ELECTRONIC HEALTH RECORDS (EHR)

- **Centralized Access to Medical History:** EHRs provide healthcare providers with immediate access to a patient's complete medical history, reducing errors and ensuring informed treatment. I was one of the first doctors to sign up to have an EMR in my office.
- **Improved Accuracy and Reduced Errors:** EHRs eliminate errors like illegible handwriting or misplaced files, enhancing the overall quality of care.
- **Enhanced Communication Between Providers:** Seamless sharing among healthcare teams ensures everyone involved in your care is on the same page.
- **Real-Time Access to Test Results and Treatment Plans:** Test results are uploaded instantly, allowing for timely diagnosis and care adjustments.

Accessing and Managing Your EHR

- **Register for Patient Portals:** Secure online platforms give access to EHRs and essential health information.
- **Navigate the EHR Interface:** Familiarize yourself with the portal's sections for test results, medications, and appointments.

- **Download and Share Medical Records**: Easily share records with specialists or new providers as needed.
- **Keep Health Information Updated**: Regularly review and update your records for accuracy.

Patient Engagement and Self-Management with EHRs

- **Track Health Metrics Over Time**: Monitor trends in blood pressure, glucose, and other vital signs.
- **Set and Monitor Health Goals**: Use EHR tools to set goals, track progress, and stay motivated.
- **Access Educational Resources**: Patient portals often offer articles and resources tailored to your needs.
- **Secure Messaging with Providers**: Conveniently ask questions or update your provider on your condition through the portal.
- **Have Your Provider Review All Results:** It is very important for your provider to go over ALL test results with you as a patient. It is not your responsibility to decipher your test results in your EHR. The prescribing doctor is trained to explain the significance of a positive test and even a negative test. Just because a test is negative does not mean it is insignificant to your general health.

Privacy and Security with EHRs

- **Understand HIPAA Regulations**: HIPAA sets strict rules for protecting your health information.
- **Use Strong Passwords and Encryption**: Regularly update passwords and use secure features on patient portals.
- **Report Suspicious Activity**: Notify your provider immediately if you notice unusual activity on your portal.

- **Securely Share Records:** Use encrypted services or portal features when sharing records with authorized providers.

HEALTH APPS AND TOOLS FOR MANAGING YOUR CARE

Health apps and tools are important in managing various aspects of healthcare. Categories of helpful health apps include:

- **Fitness and Nutrition Tracking:** Apps like MyFitnessPal and Fitbit allow you to log workouts, track calories, and monitor sleep patterns.
- **Medication Management and Reminders**: Apps like Medisafe send alerts to ensure timely medication doses and provide information on drug interactions.
- **Chronic Disease Management:** Tools like MySugr apps for diabetes or Propeller apps for asthma, to name a few, offer reminders, tracking, and resources specific to these conditions.
- **Mental Health and Mindfulness**: Apps like Headspace and Calm offer meditation, breathing exercises, and sleep aids to support mental well-being.

Choosing the Right Health Apps

- **Read User Reviews and Ratings**: By doing so, you gain insights into app usability, reliability, and effectiveness.
- **Look for Professional Endorsements:** Apps recommended by healthcare providers or organizations offer added credibility.
- **Look at Ratings:** Look for a large number of 4-5 star ratings.

Integrating Health Apps with EHRs

- **Automated Data Sharing**: Health apps connected to EHRs provide providers with real-time updates.
- **Improved Health Metrics Tracking**: Monitor trends over time and share with healthcare providers for a comprehensive health view.
- **Enhanced Coordination of Care**: Integrated health data keeps all providers informed and aligned with your health goals.
- **Facilitating Remote Monitoring and Follow-Up**: Enables ongoing monitoring of chronic conditions and allows timely treatment adjustments.

Maximizing the Use of Health Apps

- **Set Realistic Health Goals:** Goals such as weight loss, chronic condition management, or stress reduction keep you motivated.
- **Regularly Update Health Data:** Log activities, symptoms, and progress consistently to make informed health decisions.
- **Use Reminders and Notifications:** Notifications help you remember essential activities, like taking medication or exercising.
- **Engage in Community Support:** Joining challenges or sharing progress creates a supportive and accountable environment.

EMBRACING TECHNOLOGY IN YOUR HEALTHCARE JOURNEY

Health apps, EHRs, and telehealth are designed to support and enhance your healthcare experience. By choosing the right technology, integrating it effectively, and actively engaging with these tools, you can take a more proactive role in managing your health, empower yourself, and ensure you receive the best possible care. As a physician who has practiced medicine for over forty years, I have witnessed the marvelous improvement of patient care with the advancement of technology.

6

THE POWER OF PREVENTIVE SCREENINGS

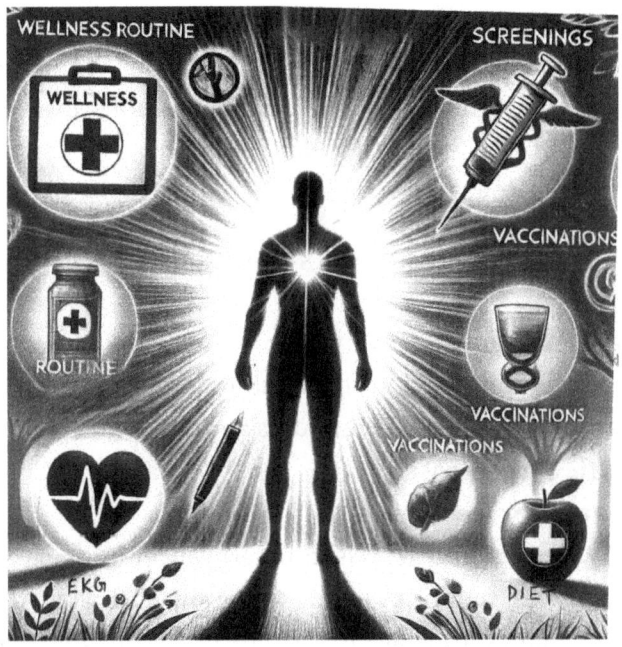

W riting this book made me think of Grace, a vibrant woman in her sixties who was my patient for thirty years. She was in politics and very intelligent but gregarious and fun. Grace was full of anecdotal knowledge, making our visits pleasant and informative. She was one of those patients we loved seeing on the schedule because she desired and understood how to maintain her health.

Grace had recently undergone a routine mammogram, which revealed early-stage breast cancer. The early detection made her treatment plan swift and effective, allowing her to return to her active lifestyle with minimal disruption. Grace's story is a powerful reminder of preventive screenings' critical role in identifying health issues before they become serious problems.

This chapter explores the various aspects of preventive care, emphasizing the importance of regular screenings and how they can significantly impact your health and well-being. The power of preventive screenings is essential in the early detection of diseases, leading to better outcomes and lower healthcare costs. Early detection allows for interventions when conditions are most treatable, often before symptoms appear.

BENEFITS OF PREVENTIVE SCREENINGS

- **Early Detection:**
  - Enables interventions for diseases at the most treatable stages, often before symptoms appear.
- **Specific Screenings:**
  - **Cancer Screenings:**
    - **Mammograms:** Detect breast cancer in its early stages, significantly increasing survival rates. This should start at age forty to forty-five in women with average risk.
    - **Colonoscopies:** These identify and remove precancerous polyps, preventing colorectal cancer.

They should start at age forty-five in patients at average risk.
- **Pap Smears and HPV Tests:** Detect abnormal cervical cells, allowing early treatment before cancer develops. Pap smears should start at age twenty-one, regardless of sexual activity. Starting at age thirty, women can begin co-testing with Pap smears and HPV tests every five years.
- Basic Cardiovascular Screenings:
  - **Cholesterol and Blood Pressure Checks:** Monitor and address hypertension and abnormal HDL and LDL cholesterol; monitoring should start at eighteen and twenty years old, respectively. Reducing heart disease and stroke risks.
- Diabetes Screenings:
  - **A1C Tests:** Assess blood sugar levels over three months, preventing complications such as neuropathy and kidney disease.
- Bone Density Tests:
  - Measure bone strength, enabling early interventions for osteoporosis to prevent fractures. This should start at age 65 y/o in patients with average risk

Screening Recommendations by Age and Risk Factors

- **Annual Physical Exams:**
  - I wish I did not have to say this, but your doctor should have you remove your clothes and give you a gown for a full PE. I am including this statement because a doctor examined me at my last annual PE in my full winter attire.
  - Provide a regular overview of health status, with

routine tests and discussions on further screenings based on age, gender, and risk factors.

- **Routine Blood Test Screenings:**
  - The frequency depends on age and health history. These screenings include CBC (blood count), CMP (blood chemistries, liver enzymes, kidney function), lipids (HDL, LDL), vitamin D levels, thyroid function (TSH, T3, T4), blood sugar (HGBA1c), and urinalysis.
- **Age-Specific Screenings:**
  - **Prostate Exams:** These include rectal and/or PSA tests for men over fifty, and for men with a high-risk (for example, black men), forty. These help detect prostate cancer early.
- **Risk-Based Screenings:**
  - **Lipoprotein A levels:** These screenings are for individuals with a family history of coronary heart disease.
  - **BRCA Gene Testing:** These are for individuals with a family history of breast cancer. These tests guide preventive strategies for high-risk individuals.

Preparing for Preventive Screenings

- **Fasting for Blood Tests:**
  - Understandingly, it is hard to do, but it is important.
  - Follow fasting instructions carefully to ensure accurate blood glucose and lipid measurements.
- **Medication Considerations:**
  - Certain drugs can affect test results, so confirm with your doctor which to pause before your screening.
- **Medical Documentation:**
  - Bring a list of your current medications and a detailed

medical history to your appointment to help interpret results accurately.

THE ROLE OF HEALTHCARE PROVIDERS

- **Scheduling and Referrals:**
  - Primary care providers (PCPs) recommend and schedule screenings based on your health profile and refer you to specialists when needed.
- **Understanding Results:**
  - Because of managed care and the recent shortage of physicians, I see patients being asked to look into patient portals on the computer to get their results. This is absurd and dangerous because patients are not equipped to interpret abnormal results and their significance. Even normal results in certain circumstances can be misconstrued. After screenings, your provider should discuss the results with you either in person or via telemedicine, or if the labs are totally normal in a patient with no risk factors, a phone call by the doctor or the RN is appropriate. Necessary lifestyle changes, further tests, or treatments may be recommended, ensuring you understand your next steps.

7

DEALING WITH INSURANCE CHALLENGES

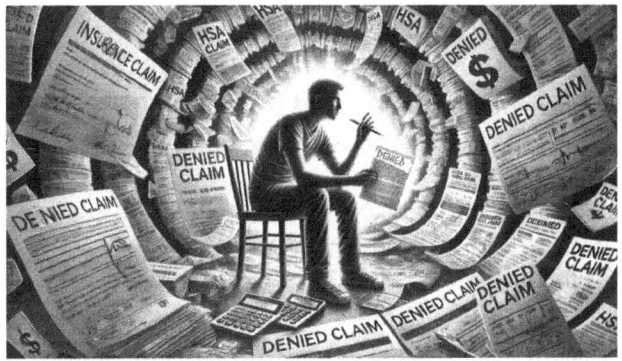

One winter, about thirteen years ago, I had a new patient who came to me because he was angry at his PCP. He was frustrated and overwhelmed because the insurance company denied coverage for the critical back surgery he needed. They recommended a noninvasive approach first, such as injections and physical therapy. In the meantime, he was still having pain. He believed his previous doctor did not try hard enough for him to get the surgery. That could have been true.

Prior authorizations are a few things some doctors do not want to do in their practice. Doing prior authorizations can be frustrating and time-consuming. Usually, insurance companies have precise things that the physician must document before they approve the procedure. If the doctor or staff didn't complete the required documentation or activity, no matter how small or seemingly insignificant, that is why the PA was denied.

YOU MUST UNDERSTAND INSURANCE DENIALS AND APPEALS

Insurance claim denials can be frustrating and occur for many reasons, and understanding these can help you address the issues effectively. One common reason is the need for prior authorization. Insurance companies often require pre-approval for specific treatments or procedures. If this step is missed, your claim may be denied. Know which services need prior authorization and ensure your healthcare provider submits the necessary documentation before proceeding.

Service Not Medically Necessary

Another reason for denial is the insurance company's determination that a service is not medically necessary. This can happen if the insurer believes the treatment is experimental, not supported by clinical guidelines, or less expensive alternatives are available, even if, unfortunately, they are not as effective. To contest this, you need to provide strong evidence, including medical records and letters from your healthcare provider, demonstrating the necessity of the treatment.

Administrative Errors

Incorrect billing codes or administrative errors are also frequent causes of claim denials. A simple mistake in coding or paperwork can lead to a denial. It's essential to carefully review the explanation of benefits (EOB) to identify errors and work with your healthcare provider to correct them. Additionally, using out-of-network providers can result in a denial if your plan does not cover services outside its network. Always confirm that your provider is in-network before receiving non-emergency care to avoid unexpected costs.

Process of Appealing Insurance Denials

When faced with a denial, the appeal process can be daunting, and the decision involves several key steps. Start by reviewing the EOB to understand the specific reason for the denial. This document outlines the insurer's justification and is your starting point for the appeal. Next, gather supporting documentation from your healthcare providers. This includes gathering medical records, test results, and letters explaining why the treatment or procedure is necessary. Detailed and comprehensive documentation will strengthen your case.

Writing a compelling appeal letter is essential. Clearly state why you believe the denial was incorrect and provide evidence to support your argument. Include your gathered documentation and reference any relevant insurance policy language or clinical guidelines. Submit your appeal within the required timeframe, typically outlined in the denial letter. Missing this deadline can forfeit your right to appeal, so timely submission is critical.

Throughout my career, I have found thorough documentation is essential throughout the appeal process. Keep copies of all correspondence with the insurance company, including emails, letters, and fax confirmations. Document phone calls and in-person conversations, noting the date, time, and names of the representatives you spoke with. Retain all medical records and bills related to the denied service. Tracking appeal submission dates and deadlines ensures you stay organized and do not miss critical steps.

Successful appeal strategies often involve submitting letters of medical necessity from your healthcare providers. These letters should detail why the treatment is essential for your condition and address any points raised in the denial. Citing relevant insurance policy language and guidelines can also support your appeal. For example, highlight this information in your appeal letter if your policy covers specific treatments under certain conditions. Utilizing state insurance commission resources can provide additional support. These agencies can offer guidance on the appeals process and may intervene on your behalf if necessary.

Checklist for Appealing Insurance Denials

1. **Review the Explanation of Benefits (EOB)**
    - Identify the reason for denial.
    - Understand the insurer's justification.
2. **Gather Supporting Documentation**
    - Collect medical records and test results.
    - Obtain letters of medical necessity from healthcare providers.
3. **Write a Compelling Appeal Letter**
    - Clearly state your argument.
    - Reference relevant policy language.
    - Include all supporting documents.
4. **Submit the Appeal Timely**
    - Adhere to the submission deadline.

- Use certified mail or a tracking service for proof of submission.
5. **Maintain Thorough Documentation**
    - Keep copies of all correspondence.
    - Document phone calls and conversations.
    - Retain medical records and bills.

Following these steps can significantly improve your chances of overturning a denial and ensuring you receive medical care.

NAVIGATING OUT-OF-POCKET COSTS AND COPAYS

Deductibles

Understanding out-of-pocket costs starts with breaking down their key components. Deductibles are the initial amounts you must pay out of your pocket before your insurance begins to cover your medical expenses. For instance, if your deductible is $1,500, you must pay for covered healthcare services before your insurance starts contributing. Deductibles can significantly impact your overall costs, especially if you have frequent medical needs. Once the deductible is met, you then move on to copayments and coinsurance.

Copayments, or Copays

Copayments, or copays, are fixed amounts you pay for specific services. These can vary depending on the type of service. For example, you might pay a $30 copay for a primary care visit and $50 for a specialist. Prescription medications also come with their own copays, which can range widely depending on whether the drug is generic or brand-name. Copays are straightforward and predictable, making budgeting for routine healthcare expenses easier.

Coinsurance

Coinsurance is a percentage of the cost of a covered healthcare service. After meeting your deductible, you might be responsible for 20 percent of the price of a service while your insurance covers the remaining 80 percent. Understanding your plan's coinsurance rate is crucial, as these percentages can add up quickly, particularly for expensive treatments or surgeries. Additionally, most insurance plans have a maximum out-of-pocket limit, which caps the total amount you must pay in a given year. Once you reach this limit, your insurance covers 100 percent of your covered services for the remainder of the year, providing a financial safety net.

In-Network Providers

Managing and reducing out-of-pocket expenses involves several practical strategies. First, always use in-network providers. These providers have negotiated rates with your insurance company, which results in lower costs for you. Before scheduling any appointments or procedures, confirm that the provider is in-network. This simple step can save you a significant amount of money.

Generic and Older Medication

Exploring generic medication options is another effective way to reduce costs. Generic and older drugs are typically much cheaper than their brand-name or newer counterparts. They may be just as effective, but many times they are not. Ask your doctor if a generic version is available when he prescribes a medication and whether the generic or older drug is as effective. Generics can be as effective, but you need to know that a generic medication can be made by different pharmaceutical companies, which can give different and sometimes subpar results. Generics can lead to substantial savings over time, especially if you're on long-term medication. However, it is important to be aware of the downsides.

Preventive Services Are Essential

Taking advantage of preventive services covered by your insurance can prevent more significant health issues down the line. Most insurance plans cover preventive services like vaccinations, screenings, and annual check-ups at no additional cost. Regularly utilizing these services can help catch potential health problems early, reducing the need for more expensive treatments later.

Other Ways of Getting Medical Expenses Paid

Negotiating payment plans with healthcare providers is another viable option. If you're facing a large medical bill, many providers are willing to set up payment plans that allow you to pay off the debt over time. This can make managing your healthcare expenses more manageable without compromising your financial stability. Don't hesitate to ask about payment options if you're struggling to pay a bill. I have always allowed some patients to be on a payment plan.

Health savings accounts (HSAs) and flexible spending accounts (FSAs) are tools designed to help manage out-of-pocket healthcare expenses. HSAs are available to individuals with high-deductible health plans (HDHPs) and allow you to contribute pre-tax dollars to an account that can be used for qualified medical expenses. One of the key benefits of HSAs is that the funds roll over year to year, and they can be invested, potentially growing your healthcare savings over time.

FSAs, on the other hand, are offered by many employers and allow you to contribute pre-tax dollars to cover eligible medical expenses. However, unlike HSAs, FSAs typically have a "use it or lose it" policy, meaning you must spend the funds within the plan year or forfeit the remaining balance. Both accounts offer tax benefits, reducing taxable income and making healthcare expenses more affordable. Maximizing account usage involves planning your contributions based on anticipated medical expenses and utilizing the funds efficiently throughout the year.

Several financial assistance programs are available to help cover out-of-pocket costs. Manufacturer assistance programs for medications often provide discounts or free medications to eligible patients who cannot afford their prescriptions. I have had patients who went directly to the pharmaceutical company and got into programs that drastically reduced the cost of their medication. These programs can be a lifeline for those on expensive medicines. Hospital financial assistance and charity care programs are designed to help patients who cannot pay their medical bills. Many hospitals offer sliding scale fees based on income; some provide free care for those in significant financial need.

Nonprofit organizations also offer grants and support for specific medical conditions. Organizations like the Leukemia & Lymphoma Society or the American Cancer Society provide financial assistance for treatment-related expenses. State and federal assistance programs for low-income individuals, such as Medicaid or Children's Health Insurance Program (CHIP), offer comprehensive coverage for those who qualify, reducing or eliminating out-of-pocket costs.

By understanding the components of out-of-pocket costs, employing strategies to manage and reduce expenses, and utilizing available financial assistance programs, you can more effectively navigate the economic aspects of your healthcare and ensure you receive the care you need without undue financial burden.

CHOOSING THE RIGHT INSURANCE PLAN FOR YOUR NEEDS: HMO, PPO, EPO, POS

Finding the right insurance plan can feel overwhelming, even for me. Breaking down the options can make the process more manageable. When evaluating different types of plans, you must understand the distinct features of HMOs, PPOs, EPOs, and POS plans.

Health maintenance organizations (HMOs) require you to choose a primary care physician (PCP) to coordinate all your care, including specialist referrals. This choice of an HMO can result in lower costs but limits you to in-network providers with a strong emphasis on cost containment.

Preferred provider organizations (PPOs) offer more flexibility, allowing you to see any doctor without a referral, including out-of-network providers, though at a higher cost.

Exclusive provider organizations (EPOs) are similar to PPOs but do not cover out-of-network care except in emergencies, combining some flexibility with cost savings. Point-of-service (POS) plans blend features of HMOs and PPOs, requiring referrals for specialists but allowing out-of-network visits at higher costs.

DEDUCTIBLES AND PREMIUMS

High-Deductible vs. Low-Deductible Plans: Which One Is Best?

Understanding the differences between high-deductible and low-deductible plans is also important. High-deductible plans generally have lower monthly premiums but higher out-of-pocket costs before insurance kicks in. These plans might be suitable if you are healthy and don't anticipate frequent medical needs.

While low-deductible plans have higher premiums, they provide more immediate coverage, which can benefit those with chronic conditions or significant medical expenses. Another critical factor is evaluating the network of providers and covered services. Ensure your preferred doctors and necessary services are included in the plan's network to avoid unexpected expenses.

High Premiums vs. Low Premiums: What's Good for One Patient May Not Be Good for All!

When considering your health needs and financial situation, aligning insurance choices with your health requirements and budget constraints is important. Assess chronic health conditions and ongoing treatment needs. For instance, if you have a chronic illness that requires regular specialist visits and medications, a plan with higher premiums but lower out-of-pocket costs might be more economical.

Estimating annual healthcare costs based on past usage can help you make an informed decision. Review your healthcare expenses over the past year to gauge your potential needs. Balancing premium costs with potential out-of-pocket expenses is a critical consideration. Lower premiums might seem attractive but could lead to higher overall costs if you need frequent medical care.

OPEN ENROLLMENT: WHAT YOU NEED TO KNOW

The open enrollment period is the designated time to enroll in or change your insurance plan each year. Critical dates for open enrollment periods are typically in the fall, but it's important to check specific dates based on your employer or marketplace. Qualifying life events like marriage, job loss, or childbirth allow for special enrollment outside the standard period. Gather all necessary information during enrollment, including your current healthcare needs, budget, and preferred providers. Resources for assistance with enrollment decisions include insurance brokers, online tools, and customer service representatives who can provide guidance tailored to your situation.

Maximizing benefits from your chosen plan involves several strategies. Preventive and wellness benefits can help you maintain your health and catch potential issues early. Most insurance plans cover preventive services such as vaccinations, screenings, and annual check-ups at no additional cost.

Another important strategy is staying within the network to minimize expenses. In-network providers have negotiated rates with your insurance, lowering out-of-pocket costs. Understanding and using annual plan benefits, including vision and dental coverage, can enhance your healthcare experience. Knowing how much the plan pays for dental and vision coverage may be essential. These benefits are often overlooked but can provide significant value.

Reviewing plan details and updates regularly ensures you are always aware of any changes in coverage, network providers, or costs. Insurance plans can change yearly, so staying informed is essential to avoid surprises. By carefully evaluating different insurance plans, aligning your choices with your health and financial needs, and fully utilizing the benefits provided, you can more effectively navigate the complexities of the managed care system.

Understanding how to select the right insurance plan and optimize its benefits will better equip you to manage your healthcare needs effectively. This knowledge will improve your health outcomes and ensure financial stability. As we move forward, we'll explore practical steps for managing chronic conditions within the managed care system, ensuring you receive comprehensive and coordinated care.

Navigating the open enrollment period for health insurance can be challenging. Fortunately, Here are a few examples of where you can go to aid in the enrollment of insurance plans:

1. **HealthCare.gov**: The official health insurance marketplace for the United States, HealthCare.gov, allows users to compare and enroll in health insurance plans. Additionally, it offers a "Find Local Help" feature to locate in-person assistance.
2. **State-Based Marketplaces:** Many states operate their own health insurance marketplaces. For instance, New Jersey residents can use GetCoveredNJ to explore and enroll in coverage options. These platforms often provide tailored resources and assistance dependent on the state's offerings.
3. **HealthSherpa:** An alternative to HealthCare.gov, HealthSherpa is a private platform that enables users to compare ACA-compliant health insurance plans and determine their subsidy eligibility. It offers a streamlined enrollment process and access to licensed agents.

4. **eHealthInsurance:** This online marketplace allows individuals to compare health insurance plans from various carriers. eHealthInsurance provides tools to filter plans based on preferences and needs.
5. **GoHealth:** GoHealth operates an online health insurance marketplace offering individual health insurance and short-term health insurance. It provides tools to help users compare plans.
6. **State Health Insurance Assistance Programs (SHIPs):** These programs offer free local counseling to Medicare beneficiaries and their families. They help beneficiaries understand benefits, coverage options, and enrollment processes.
7. **CMS Partner Tools & Toolkits:** The Centers for Medicare & Medicaid Services (CMS) offers educational materials and resources to promote and assist consumers in enrolling in the Marketplace.
8. **Navigator Programs:** Funded by federal or state grants, navigators and assisters provide free, unbiased assistance to consumers exploring health insurance options. They can help with understanding plan details, eligibility criteria, and the enrollment process.

8

CASE STUDIES AND REAL-LIFE SCENARIOS—INFORMATION PROVIDED TO ME BY NEW OR ESTABLISHED PATIENTS WHO HAD CONFLICTS WITH SPECIALISTS

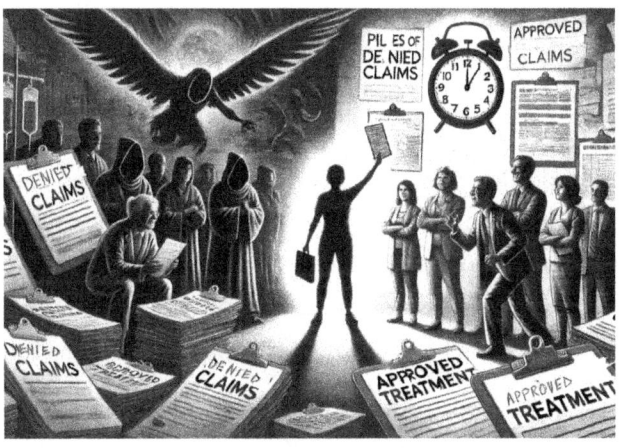

About seven to eight years ago, I had a new patient named Karen, who had been battling severe arthritis for years. Her condition had deteriorated to the point where everyday activities became excruciatingly painful. To make matters worse, Karen was newly reunited with her first-year-college love, Bobby, after being a widow for ten years. Bobby was active and vibrant, and the last thing she wanted him to see was her disability. But there was hope.

Karen told me her rheumatologist recommended a new, advanced medication that promised significant relief.

However, her insurance company denied the initial prior authorization request, citing cost concerns. This setback devastated Karen, who had pinned her hopes on this treatment. After months of going back and forth with her insurance company's prior authorization department, we finally got her treatment. Her story speaks to the hurdles my patients faced along with many others in the managed care system and the importance of persistence and effective communication in overcoming these challenges.

OVERCOMING PRIOR AUTHORIZATION DELAYS

Karen's severe arthritis had reached a critical point. Traditional treatments were no longer effective, and her rheumatologist recommended an advanced biologic medication. Though promising, this treatment came with a hefty price tag, making insurance approval essential. The initial denial from Karen's insurance company was a significant blow. The insurer argued that the medication was too expensive and suggested alternatives that Karen stated she had already tried without success. This denial set the stage for a protracted battle to secure the necessary treatment.

The first step in the fight was comprehensive documentation of medical necessity. Karen told me she appreciated the rheumatologist's role in this part of her journey. She meticulously detailed Karen's medical history, previous treatments, and their ineffectiveness. The documentation included extensive medical records, test results, and a compelling letter from the rheumatologist explaining why the advanced medication was necessary. This letter highlighted the progressive nature of Karen's arthritis and the failure of conventional treatments, making a strong case for the necessity of biological medication.

Karen and I began making frequent follow-up calls to the insurance company as a daily routine. Each call aimed to check the status of the prior authorization request, address any additional queries the insurer had, and ensure that the case remained a priority. Karen also enlisted the help of a patient advocate, a professional experienced in navigating the complexities of insurance approvals. The advocate's expertise was invaluable, providing guidance on the appeals process and helping to streamline communication between Karen, her healthcare provider, and the insurance company.

Effective communication and persistence were the cornerstones of Karen's eventual success. Regular updates between Karen, myself, and her rheumatologist ensured that all parties were on the same page. The rheumatologist provided clear and concise explanations of Karen's condition and the benefits of the advanced medication during every interaction with the insurance company. This transparency and consistency helped to build a compelling case that was difficult to ignore. The patient advocate also played a role in maintaining consistent communication, ensuring that no detail was overlooked and that every piece of evidence was presented.

After weeks of relentless effort, the breakthrough came. The insurance company finally approved the medication, recognizing the comprehensive evidence of its necessity. The approval marked a significant victory for Karen, who soon began her new treatment. The advanced medication brought substantial relief, improving her quality of life and allowing her to resume activities she had long abandoned. The treatment also allowed her to resume a relationship with a healthy suitor from her past, which was icing on the cake. This case underscores the importance of being proactive and persistent when dealing with prior authorization issues. Karen's experience illustrates that while the process can be arduous, effective communication and a well-documented case can lead to a successful outcome.

REFLECTION SECTION: STRATEGIES FOR OVERCOMING PRIOR AUTHORIZATION DELAYS

- **Gather Comprehensive Documentation:** Ensure all medical records, test results, and a detailed letter of medical necessity from your healthcare provider are included.
- **Frequent Follow-Up Calls**: Regularly check the status of your prior authorization request and promptly address any additional queries.
- **Involve a Patient Advocate:** This advocate can be a well-informed, articulate friend or family member. You should also seek the help of a professional advocate to navigate the complexities of insurance approvals.
- **Maintain Effective Communication:** Keep all parties informed with regular updates and clear, concise explanations of your condition and treatment benefits.

Karen's journey from initial denial to eventual approval is a powerful example of the challenges and triumphs of navigating the managed care system. Her story highlights the critical role of persistence, effective communication, and comprehensive documentation in securing necessary medical treatments.

EFFECTIVE SELF-ADVOCACY IN A HOSPITAL SETTING

About ten years ago, I encountered a new patient in my practice; let's call him Jim. I am going to surmise the history he gave me. Jim stated he was admitted for a severe respiratory infection by his last doctor. Jim's condition was critical, and he required intensive treatment to stabilize. Despite his serious state, hospital cost-cutting measures threatened to discharge him prematurely. Aware of the risks, Jim told me he decided to take an active role in his care to ensure he received appropriate treatment.

Jim's first step was to request detailed explanations of his treatment plans and discharge criteria. Jim intentionally spoke to his doctors, asking them to outline his diagnosis, the planned interventions, and the specific criteria they would use to determine when he was ready for discharge. This information was necessary for Jim to understand what to expect and gauge whether the proposed timeline was realistic. By insisting on clarity, Jim ensured his care team was accountable and transparent, providing a solid foundation for his self-advocacy efforts.

Involving a family member in discussions with healthcare providers proved invaluable for Jim. His sister, a retired nurse, attended meetings with doctors, helping him ask pertinent questions and take notes. Her medical background allowed her to understand complex medical jargon and advocate effectively on Jim's behalf. This collaboration ensured that Jim's concerns were addressed comprehensively and he had support in making informed decisions about his care. Having a family member present also provided emotional support, reducing the stress and anxiety associated with his hospitalization.

Jim meticulously documented his symptoms and treatment responses, noting every change in his condition, medication administered, and new symptoms. This record was helpful to his doctors, empowering him to track his progress and identify any discrepancies in his treatment plan. By maintaining this log, Jim could provide his healthcare team with accurate updates, ensuring they had the most current and comprehensive information to inform their decisions.

As concerns about his impending discharge grew, Jim requested a second opinion from a specialist. He requested a consultation with a pulmonologist he looked up to, who thoroughly reviewed his case. The specialist confirmed that Jim was not ready for discharge, citing specific medical reasons that warranted extended care. This second opinion provided additional weight to Jim's argument, making it harder for the hospital to justify an early discharge. The specialist's input was critical in ensuring that Jim received the necessary care to fully stabilize before leaving the hospital.

Understanding his patient rights and hospital policies was a cornerstone of Jim's effective self-advocacy. He cited his right to a safe and appropriate discharge, emphasizing that premature release could jeopardize his health. Jim's knowledge of his rights gave him the confidence to challenge decisions driven by cost-cutting rather than medical necessity. He also utilized hospital patient advocacy services, enlisting the help of a patient advocate who supported his case. The advocate facilitated communication between Jim and the hospital administration, ensuring his voice was heard and his concerns were taken seriously.

The outcome of Jim's proactive approach was that he received extended care until he was fully stabilized. His persistence and clear communication with healthcare providers ensured that financial considerations did not compromise his treatment. Jim's experience underscores the importance of understanding patient rights and hospital policies, as well as the value of assertiveness and effective communication in advocating for one's own health. Jim successfully navigated a challenging situation by taking control of his care, ensuring that his doctors prioritized his health and well-being.

Jim's case teaches us that being informed and proactive can significantly impact the quality of care received in hospital settings. Understanding your rights, involving knowledgeable family members, keeping detailed records, and seeking second opinions when necessary are all strategies that can help you advocate effectively for your health. Jim's story speaks to the power of self-advocacy and the positive outcomes it can achieve.

In contrast to Jim's story, I would like to tell about another patient of mine quickly; let's call her Ruby. Ruby was an uncontrolled diabetic who was about sixty years old. Ruby entered my office, and I tested her blood sugar above 600. I immediately admitted her to the hospital, first being seen in the ER, which did more testing. She was admitted to the floor and was treated with IV fluids, medications, and insulin. I frequently called the floor to check on her. I called this time because her blood sugar was 500 on the EMR (electronic medical record) in my office, and I was following up on her lab results. I was going to adjust her insulin, but I was told by a nurse at the nursing station that I had discharged her.

At that time, I had temporarily lost my mind. I told the nurse I did not discharge her! I asked the nurse if I could speak to the patient and for her to page the nurse caring for Ruby. The nurse put me on hold for two minutes, then picked up and said the patient was no longer there. I spoke to the nurse caring for Ruby, trying to keep my composure while talking to her. She told me that someone in the administration told her the patient needed to be discharged. A nurse cannot independently discharge a patient; only a doctor can. A nurse can write the order under a doctor's instruction, so she took orders from someone in administration. I reported the nurse; she was someone I had worked with for years and believed to be a good nurse, But what she did was inexcusable. The nurse was reprimanded and disciplined.

The care team working with the administration carries themselves with much authority, often intimidating nurses and even some inexperienced doctors. In Ruby's case, I called her home and had her family bring her back to the hospital, and she was readmitted immediately. Unfortunately, Ruby did not know how to self-advocate. She knew her blood sugar was dangerously high but was afraid to stand up for herself. Ruby could have insisted on talking to me or getting a second opinion if she believed the discharge order came from me. But, she just did what she was told, which could have cost her her life.

MANAGING CHRONIC CONDITIONS IN MANAGED CARE

Consider the case of Ben, a middle-aged man diagnosed with Type 2 diabetes. Who was a patient of mine for many years? Managing his condition required regular monitoring, medication adjustments, and frequent visits to specialists. Ben faced the challenge of juggling multiple medications and coordinating appointments with various healthcare providers. For example, he frequently visited an endocrinologist, an ophthalmologist, a neurologist, a podiatrist, and a urologist. The complexity of his condition made it essential to navigate the managed care system (MCS) effectively to ensure comprehensive care.

The first step was establishing a strong relationship with me, his primary care provider (PCP). I became the cornerstone of his healthcare management, overseeing all aspects of his treatment. Our relationship was built on trust and regular communication. I took the time to understand his medical history, current condition, and treatment goals. We scheduled regular check-ups to monitor his blood glucose levels and adjust medications as needed. Our ongoing collaboration ensured Ben's care was consistent and tailored to his needs.

Utilizing a care coordinator was another strategy that significantly improved Ben's healthcare management. The care coordinator acted as a liaison between Ben, myself, and his various healthcare providers, ensuring that all appointments were scheduled efficiently and communication between specialists was streamlined. As a care coordinator, this role was particularly important when Ben needed to see an endocrinologist, podiatrist, and nutritionist regularly. The care coordinator managed these appointments, reducing the burden on Ben and ensuring that all providers were on the same page regarding his treatment plan.

Regularly updating and reviewing electronic health records (EHR) was vital in managing Ben's condition. EHRs provided a centralized and accessible platform for all his medical information. Ben's healthcare providers could easily access his records, review past treatments, and make informed decisions about his care. This seamless information sharing reduced the risk of errors and ensured that everyone involved in Ben's care had the most up-to-date information. Moreover, the EHR system allowed for quick adjustments to his treatment plan based on the latest data, enhancing the overall quality of care.

Ben also used a medication management app to track his dosages and refill schedules. Managing multiple medications can be daunting, but the app provided reminders for when to take each medication and when to order refills. This tool helped Ben stay on top of his medication regimen, reducing the risk of missed doses or running out of essential medications. The app also allowed him to track any side effects and communicate this information to his healthcare providers, enabling them to make necessary adjustments promptly.

Patient education and self-management were critical components of Ben's successful management of his Type 2 diabetes. He attended diabetes education classes where he learned about the importance of diet, exercise, and monitoring blood glucose levels. These classes gave him the knowledge and skills to manage his condition effectively. Implementing lifestyle changes, such as adopting a balanced diet and incorporating regular physical activity, significantly impacted his health. Ben also kept a health journal to record his daily blood glucose levels, meals, physical activity, and any symptoms he experienced. He brought his journal at every visit with me. This journal became a valuable tool for me to identify patterns and make informed decisions about his care.

For a short time, Ben was enrolled in our support group for chronically ill patients,Dr. D Egan (a Natropath and Functional Nutritionist) and myself gave group biweekly meetings for our patients for years The group offered Ben emotional support and practical advice from others facing similar challenges. Sharing experiences and learning from others helped him stay motivated and adhere to his treatment plan. The support group also provided a sense of community, reducing the isolation often associated with managing a chronic condition.

The outcome of these combined efforts was remarkable. Ben's blood glucose levels stabilized, and his overall health improved significantly. He experienced fewer complications and hospital visits, demonstrating the effectiveness of proactive management and continuous education in chronic care. Ben's case highlights the importance of being informed and proactive in managing chronic conditions within the managed care system. Establishing strong relationships with healthcare providers, utilizing care coordinators and digital tools, and engaging in continuous education and self-management can lead to better health outcomes and an improved quality of life.

BEN'S STORY IS ATYPICAL BUT CAN BE ACHIEVED

Unfortunately, Ben's story isn't typical. Many obstacles prevent patients from receiving this comprehensive approach to care. Patient education and the willingness of health professionals to participate in this approach can dramatically improve the outcomes for chronically ill patients.

Ben's success in managing his Type 2 diabetes underscores the importance of a coordinated and informed approach to chronic care. By leveraging the resources and support available within the managed care system, patients can effectively navigate the complexities of their conditions, leading to better health outcomes and a higher quality of life. As we transition to the next chapter, we will explore how the COVID-19 pandemic has further complicated healthcare delivery and what steps can be taken to mitigate its impact on patient care.

MAKE A DIFFERENCE WITH YOUR REVIEW

UNLOCK THE POWER OF GENEROSITY

"The best way to find yourself is to lose yourself in the service of others."

— MAHATMA GANDHI

People who give without expecting anything in return often live the most meaningful lives. Let's create real change—together.

Are you someone who wants to understand how to navigate our broken healthcare system—but didn't know where to start?

My mission with The Ultimate Handbook is to make navigating the managed care system understandable, personal, and empow

But to reach more readers, I need your help.

Most people choose books based on reviews. Will you take a moment to help another patient or caregiver who is scared, overw

It's completely free and takes just a minute, but your review could:

- Help one more patient demand a second opinion that saves their life
- Help one more family understand the power of medical advocacy
- Help one more cancer patient like June know they're not alone
- Help push the conversation on healthcare reform forward

To make a difference, please scan the QR code below or visit:

https://www.amazon.com/review/review-your-purchases/?asin=BOOKASIN

If helping others resonates with you—you're my kind of reader. Thank you from the bottom of my heart.

— Dr. Robin Snead

9

THE IMPACT OF COVID-19 ON MANAGED CARE

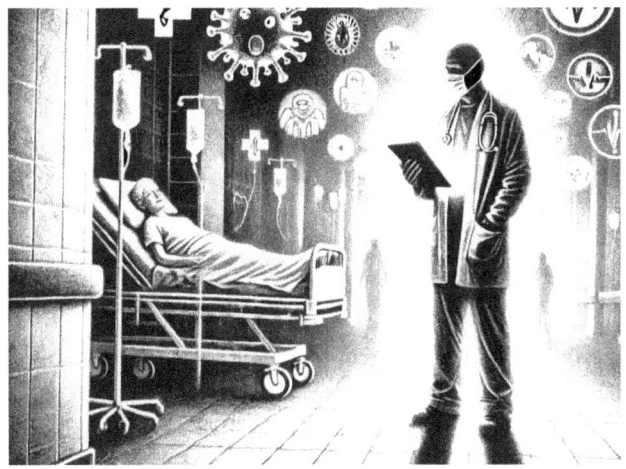

On a bright afternoon in March 2020, a young nurse named Emily who was a patient of mine walked into her usual shift in the intensive care unit (ICU), unaware that her world—and the entire healthcare landscape—was about to be turned upside down. It was just the beginning of the COVID-19 pandemic, and by the end of her shift, the hospital was flooded with COVID-19 patients, each one sicker than the last. The ICU was at capacity, every bed taken, and patients were isolated, suffering alone, and restricted from visitation.

Emily and her colleagues were running on fumes, both mentally and physically. ICU doctors and nurses were devastated. They were fearful for their lives and the lives of their loved ones at home. Emily was apprehensive about bringing this virus home to her husband and children, all of whom had asthma. Like so many others, Emily's story highlights how profoundly COVID-19 reshaped healthcare, placing unprecedented strain on the people and systems designed to protect our health.

COVID-19 AND THE EXODUS OF HEALTHCARE WORKERS

The pandemic created a perfect storm, leading to an exodus of healthcare professionals across the globe. Many left not because they wanted to but because the weight of relentless shifts and emotional strain made it nearly impossible to stay. Imagine working double shifts for weeks, each day filled with the fear of contracting a highly contagious virus and the sadness of watching patients slip away, often without loved ones by their side. Burnout, an issue healthcare workers already knew all too well, became a widespread crisis. The pandemic demanded resilience, but after months of relentless pressure, even the most dedicated nurses, doctors, and support staff began to crumble.

The shortages were further worsened by another painful reality: a scarcity of personal protective equipment (PPE). For months, many healthcare workers lacked the essential masks and gloves to feel safe, forcing them to reuse single-use masks or improvise with their own. The very people saving lives were constantly at risk of becoming patients themselves. Understandably, many began to reconsider their careers, opting to leave for the safety of their families and health.

DEATHS OF HEALTH CARE WORKERS (HCWS) AND THE END OF PRACTICING MEDICINE

The World Health Organization (WHO) estimated that between January 2020 and May 2021, approximately 80,000 to 180,000 HCWs died due to COVID-19, with a midpoint of 115,000 deaths. (WHO, 2021) In the USA, as of July 2020, the CDC reported 641 deaths among HCWs with confirmed COVID-19 (CDC, 2020). A subsequent study analyzing data up to October 2021 identified 1,469 deaths among HCWs in the US (Lin et al. 2021).

Financial strain also became an inescapable issue for those of us in private practice. With restrictions on office visits, many practices, including mine, which I have owned for over thirty-five years, couldn't sustain themselves under the new limitations. Healthcare, typically known for its stability, had become as uncertain as any other field. Clinics closed, hours were cut, and job security—once a given—felt precarious.

IMPACT ON PATIENT CARE: A RIPPLE EFFECT

The shortage of healthcare professionals rippled across the system, affecting patient care in every conceivable way. Longer wait times became the norm as the remaining workforce struggled to meet demand. Patients suddenly found themselves waiting weeks or months for appointments that once required a mere phone call. And these delays weren't just an inconvenience; they were often life-altering. Cardiovascular patients face increased mortality risk due to delayed hospital visits. Regarding healthcare, timeliness can distinguish between early detection, missed diagnosis, or a full-blown crisis.

Those who remained in healthcare faced increased workloads, which compounded the issue. The irony was impossible to ignore: Healthcare professionals were burning out faster by working harder, worsening the shortages. Overwhelmed and exhausted, these providers needed help delivering the quality of care they were trained to give. Errors increased, patient safety became a concern, and the entire system strained under the weight of too many patients and too few providers.

MY PERSONAL EXPERIENCE AS A PATIENT

One evening, I was preparing for bed and brushing my teeth when I started having mild pain in my left scapula. It did not go away. I chewed up six 81 mg aspirins and called 911. I was taken to the nearest hospital, which was close, where I signed in and told the front desk I was having left scapula pain that could be cardiac. Occasionally, the pain felt like it radiated to my left chest. I did not have difficulty breathing. They took me in, took my vital signs, and had me sit in the ER waiting room. I sat there for nine hours, even telling two nurses at separate times that my chest pain was getting worse. They did nothing.

After nine hours, I asked the front desk why it had taken so long to be seen. I reiterated my age and said I once had cardiac problems thirty-five years ago that had resolved. I even stooped, out of desperation, to tell the front desk I was a doctor who graduated from their medical school. This exclamation made absolutely no difference. The waiting room was packed. I asked the nurse at the front desk why is it so busy, and she told me it was because of the unvaccinated COVID patients. After ten-plus hours, a nurse took me to the back, where I was examined, had blood work, and was put on a stress test machine. My blood test, ECG, stress test, and echo, all done in the ER, were negative. This was in early 2021, and the ERs were still flooded with patients with COVID-19.

COVID-19 CAUSED PROBLEMS FOR OTHER NON-COVID-19 PATIENTS WITH ACUTE AND CHRONIC DISEASES

One study reported a significant decline (43 percent) in hospitalizations for acute cardiovascular conditions in March 2020 compared to March 2019. In the United States, even in children, asthma admissions saw a similar decline (Bratt et al. 2020).

Healthcare systems prioritized COVID-19 care, leading to deferred treatments for other chronic and acute conditions. Hospitals experienced shortages of critical resources, including intensive care beds and staff, further impacting care availability for non-COVID patients.

The surge in COVID-19 cases, particularly among unvaccinated patients, caused significant delays in emergency treatment for acute non-COVID conditions. For example, delays in treating exacerbations of chronic diseases like asthma and COPD were due to the prioritization of COVID-19 cases (Watson et al. 2021).

The impact was particularly harsh in specialized care. With fewer specialists, patients with chronic or complex conditions found it increasingly difficult to access the needed expertise. It was a time of deep frustration and, in many cases, growing despair.

TEMPORARY AND TRAVELING HEALTHCARE WORKERS: THE STOPGAP SOLUTION

Managed care organizations turned to temporary and traveling healthcare workers as a stopgap. These professionals were brought in from other regions or hired for short-term contracts, which helped fill immediate gaps. However, it came with challenges. Continuity of care suffered as rotating providers treated patients, each new to their medical history and needs. For permanent staff, integrating these temporary workers into their routines wasn't always seamless; it added complexity to an already demanding job.

Expanding the roles of nurse practitioners (NPs) and physician assistants (PAs) also became essential. These professionals are skilled, highly trained, and essential to the healthcare system. However, there was some tension. Some physicians felt that supervising NPs and PAs added to their workload, while others worried that the complexities of certain cases went beyond the training of NPs and PAs. Still, their contribution was invaluable; by handling routine cases and preventive care, NPs and PAs freed doctors to focus on more critical needs.

TELEHEALTH: HEALTHCARE'S NEW FRONTIER

If there was one silver lining in this upheaval, it was the rapid rise of telehealth. Practically overnight, telehealth went from a niche service to an essential tool in patient care. For patients, telehealth meant they could consult with their doctors from the safety of their own homes, avoiding crowded waiting rooms and minimizing exposure. For healthcare providers, it allowed them to see more patients in less time, reducing some of the pressures on physical facilities.

Telehealth proved invaluable for routine follow-ups, mental health services, and chronic condition management. Patients could check in with their doctors about minor ailments or discuss test results without the hassle of commuting. For those dealing with mental health issues, the ability to connect virtually was a game-changer, especially as the pandemic brought its own wave of anxiety and depression.

However, as with any new approach, telehealth had its quirks. Technical issues became a common hurdle—high-speed internet wasn't universal, and not everyone could access a smartphone or computer. Privacy concerns also emerged as some were worried about the confidentiality of their virtual visits. And, of course, certain conditions require a hands-on assessment, which telehealth can't provide. Despite these limitations, telehealth became a lifeline, bridging the gap during one of the most challenging times in modern healthcare.

PRACTICAL TIPS FOR PATIENTS: NAVIGATING CARE IN A CHANGED WORLD

For patients, navigating healthcare during the pandemic has meant being flexible and adaptable. Here are some practical tips:

- **Be Flexible with Appointments:** Availability may vary, so be open to different times or seeing various providers within your network.
- **Utilize Telehealth:** Opt for virtual consultations when possible to reduce in-person visits.
- **Use Urgent Care for Non-Emergencies:** Urgent care centers can offer timely care without burdening hospitals for minor issues.

- **Build a Strong Relationship with Your PCP:** A primary care provider who knows your history can help coordinate your care and prioritize your health needs.

Managing Delays and Disruptions in Care

As ICUs filled up, hospitals were forced to prioritize COVID-19 patients, pushing back elective surgeries and routine check-ups. Unfortunately, this meant that patients with chronic conditions missed critical appointments, causing many to see their health decline. Even routine screenings, vital for early detection of serious illnesses, were postponed, potentially leading to more advanced and harder-to-treat cases in the future.

Patients who relied on regular medication faced unexpected shortages, and managing these disruptions required adaptability.

Some Ways to Handle These Challenges

- **Keep Up with Preventive Care:** Monitor your health at home, whether tracking blood pressure, checking blood sugar levels, or using other home devices. Remind your doctor of any preventive care you need that was overlooked.
- **Use Telehealth for Follow-Ups:** Opt for virtual appointments to avoid delays, but some follow-up visits require seeing a doctor in person. Barring a needed exam or physical contact, Telemedicine is an excellent choice.
- **Prioritize Urgent Needs:** Work with your healthcare provider to identify what can't be postponed, ensuring essential care isn't overlooked.
- **Stay Informed and Proactive:** Reach out to your providers, ask about alternatives if needed, and stay

updated on healthcare services and policies that may impact your care.

The pandemic reshaped healthcare in ways we're still adapting to. While it's been challenging, it has also shown the resilience and adaptability of healthcare workers and patients alike. By staying informed, proactive, and flexible, we can continue to navigate these changes and ensure our health remains a priority—even in the most unprecedented times.

10

ADDRESSING IATROGENIC DEATHS AND MEDICAL ERRORS

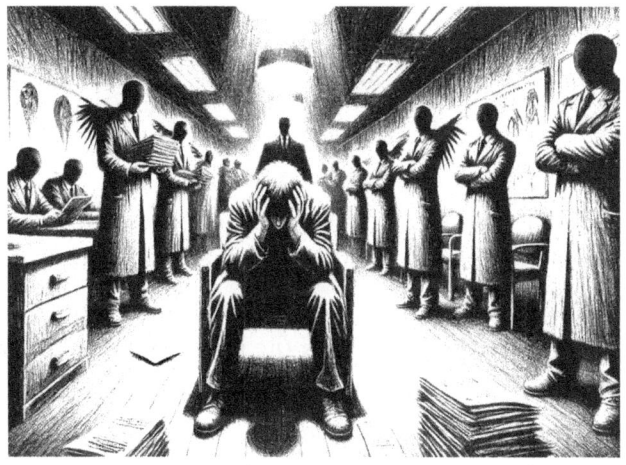

One late evening, I received a call no doctor ever wanted to take. The voice on the other end belonged to the widow of a past patient, Peter, who I had not seen in several years. I had a relationship with them because they had been patients of mine for ten years before they moved to a different state. Peter had been admitted for what should have been a straightforward, routine procedure. But a string of errors—a misdiagnosis, a medication mix-up, and a hospital-acquired infection—had led to a tragic outcome. Peter's widow insisted that Peter's care was treated haphazardly. Peter's death really bothered me, not only because he was once my patient but because it is a powerful, personal reminder of the severe risks that accompany medical care in a world where errors, oversights, and system failures can and do occur.

Peter's story is far from unique. It illustrates the genuine, often overlooked dangers of iatrogenic deaths—deaths caused by the medical treatment process itself, including errors, infections, and adverse reactions to drugs. These types of fatalities reveal the vulnerabilities within our healthcare system and the urgent need for change to prioritize patient safety.

UNDERSTANDING IATROGENIC DEATHS: A GROWING CRISIS

"Iatrogenic" deaths—those resulting from the care process itself—have become a significant issue in modern healthcare. In the United States alone, roughly 400,000 hospitalized patients experience preventable harm each year (*Journal of Patient Safety*, James 2013). medical errors now rank as the third leading cause of death in the US, just behind heart disease and cancer, surpassing accidents and strokes per a 2016 article in the BMJ (Makary & Daniel 2016). This statistic highlights a troubling reality: the healthcare system designed to protect us sometimes fails, with life-altering consequences.

The factors behind these errors are complex. Misdiagnoses, surgical mistakes, and hospital-acquired infections (HAIs) top the list. Imagine a patient misdiagnosed with a minor ailment who doesn't receive prompt treatment for a much more serious, underlying condition or consider the impact of a wrong-site surgery.

Hospital-acquired infections, often due to lapses in hygiene or contaminated equipment, also claim lives—particularly among those with weakened immune systems. Medication errors, from incorrect dosages to harmful drug interactions, further complicate matters, while systemic issues like understaffing and insufficient training create an environment where mistakes are more likely.

PROBLEMS OF LESS EXPERIENCED NPS, PAS, AND OVERWORKED PHYSICIANS

Ironically, managed care systems—designed to control healthcare costs—can sometimes increase the risk of these tragedies. Tight budgets and rushed procedures can prompt providers to cut corners. For instance, a surgeon under pressure to perform back-to-back procedures might skip a safety check. Early discharges, meant to reduce hospital costs, can backfire if patients aren't fully stabilized.

Furthermore, managed care often relies on less experienced healthcare providers (NPs and PAs) or overworked healthcare providers to keep costs down. These providers, while competent, may lack the expertise or energy to manage complex cases effectively, leading to higher error rates. I have been a collaborative physician in several companies and allowed NPs to do medical rotations in my office. From what I have witnessed, NPs and PAs typically do a good job with uncomplicated routine cases. Also, there have been quite a few questions asked by NPs and PAs that they should have known or, if not, should have known how to retrieve the answer quickly. I did help train an NP who had a doctorate. Her knowledge and ability to research things she did not know was excellent.

THE HUMAN AND ECONOMIC COST OF MEDICAL ERRORS

The toll of iatrogenic deaths is felt deeply by families and communities. For loved ones, the sudden and preventable loss is devastating. Families wrestle with grief, anger, and often a lengthy legal battle. At the same time, healthcare providers involved in these errors frequently experience guilt, depression, and self-doubt, which can affect their future performance and, in turn, patient care.

Financially, these errors place a heavy burden on the healthcare system. Treating hospital-acquired infections alone adds an estimated $45 billion to annual healthcare expenses. Malpractice suits further strain already stretched resources, diverting funds that could be used to improve patient care.

PREVENTING MEDICAL ERRORS: STRATEGIES FOR SAFER CARE

The first step in addressing iatrogenic deaths is understanding their causes. However, we must also implement proactive strategies to prevent errors and enhance patient safety.

Implementing Non-Punitive Error Reporting Systems

Creating a non-punitive culture around error reporting is essential. When healthcare professionals feel safe reporting mistakes without fear of retribution, it creates transparency and allows for a clearer view of recurring issues. Many institutions use incident reporting systems to collect error data, followed by root cause analysis (RCA) to identify underlying problems. By reviewing and updating protocols regularly, healthcare organizations can address these issues head-on, reducing the likelihood of future errors.

Continuous Education and Training

Medical knowledge and technology are constantly evolving. To keep up, healthcare providers need ongoing training on the latest tools, techniques, and procedures. Simulation-based training offers a safe environment to practice complex scenarios, allowing professionals to refine their skills without risk to patients. Emphasizing teamwork and communication in training sessions helps providers collaborate effectively, reducing the risk of miscommunication.

Medication Safety Protocols

Medication errors are a significant cause of iatrogenic deaths, but technology offers promising solutions. Electronic prescribing and barcode scanning reduce the risk of human error in medication administration. Standardized labeling and storage practices minimize mix-ups, while regular medication reconciliation during patient transitions (like hospital admissions or discharges) ensures accurate, up-to-date lists that prevent dangerous interactions.

Strict Adherence to Infection Control Practices

Preventing hospital-acquired infections is critical. Simple measures like hand hygiene, personal protective equipment (PPE), and strict cleaning protocols can significantly reduce infection rates. Regular disinfection of medical equipment and isolation procedures for infectious patients help prevent the spread of infections and protect patients and staff.

PATIENT SAFETY: WHAT YOU CAN DO TO PROTECT YOURSELF

Patients play an essential role in their safety. By staying informed and proactive, you can reduce your risk of medical errors and advocate for your health.

Educate Yourself

Knowledge is power. Research your condition, understand your treatment options, and familiarize yourself with the potential risks and benefits. Reputable sites like the Mayo Clinic and the National Institutes of Health (NIH) offer reliable information.

In addition, ways of educating yourself are expanding because of artificial intelligence (AI). A scientific app within ChatGPT called Consensus can give you some quick answers to some medical questions. It is good to lead you in the right direction for further clarification. Don't hesitate to seek second opinions if you think a proposed treatment or diagnosis is possibly wrong.

Be Active in Your Care

Bring a list of questions to appointments, and confirm details about your treatments or medications. Double-check names and dosages, and always keep a list of your current medications and any allergies. Don't be afraid to speak up if something doesn't seem right.

Use Safety Checklists and Tools

Patient safety checklists, like before surgery, can help prevent errors. Medication management apps can track prescriptions and set dose reminders. Hospital discharge checklists ensure you understand your post-discharge instructions, reducing the risk of complications. Accessing your health information through patient portals allows you to stay informed and verify the accuracy of your medical records.

Build a Support Network: An Advocate

Bringing a family member or friend to appointments provides an extra set of eyes and ears. An advocate can help you remember instructions, ask questions, and support your decisions. Having someone double-check your medications and follow-up care instructions can catch errors you might miss. A trusted support network adds practical and emotional strength, helping you navigate the healthcare system more safely.

FINAL THOUGHTS

In summary, protecting yourself from medical errors involves multiple proactive steps. By educating yourself, actively participating in your care, utilizing safety checklists and tools, and building a supportive network, you can significantly enhance your safety within the healthcare system. These strategies reduce the risk of errors and empower you to take control of your health, leading to better outcomes and greater peace of mind.

11

ENHANCING DOCTOR-PATIENT RELATIONSHIPS

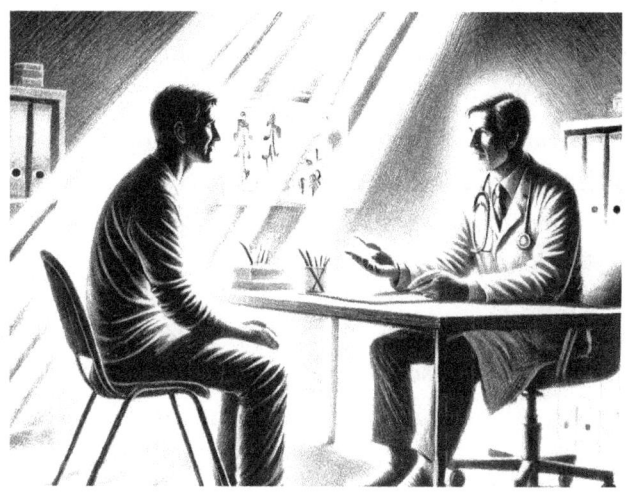

BUILDING TRUST WITH YOUR PRIMARY CARE PROVIDER

I have been practicing medicine since 1983. I have always loved practicing and appreciated patients who understood the importance of having a relationship with me. I enjoyed working with patients who showed an interest in their healthcare. These patients consistently kept their appointments and adhered to their scheduled examinations. They understood the importance of preventive screenings, kept up with the ones they were due for, and showed an interest in the results.

The consultations with these patients were productive, and their treatment was usually more effective. On my part, I treated every patient with respect, and I knew it was my responsibility to do as much as I could to cure, relieve, or make better any negative symptom or disease they have. My close relationships with many patients came from having similar goals and mutual respect.

TRUST CAN HAVE A PROFOUND IMPACT ON THE DOCTOR-PATIENT RELATIONSHIP

Establishing and maintaining trust with your PCP requires effort from both parties. Consistency in attending scheduled appointments is fundamental. Regular visits help your PCP understand your health history and detect changes early. Being honest about your symptoms, lifestyle, and challenges is equally important.

Your PCP relies on accurate information to make informed decisions about your care. Downplaying or exaggerating your symptoms can lead to misdiagnoses or inappropriate treatments. Following through on agreed-upon treatment plans demonstrates your commitment to your health and respect for your provider's expertise.

It is also essential to provide feedback on treatments and care received. If a particular medication or therapy isn't working, discuss it with your PCP. This feedback enables adjustments that better meet your needs.

Empathy and active listening play crucial roles in fostering a strong doctor-patient relationship. When both you and your PCP show genuine concern for each other's well-being, it establishes a deeper connection and understanding. For instance, if your PCP takes the time to listen without interrupting, it shows that they value your input and are committed to addressing your concerns. Similarly, acknowledging each other's perspectives and feelings can bridge gaps and prevent misunderstandings. Empathy from your primary care physician (PCP) reassures you that they are invested in your health, while your empathy toward them fosters a respectful and cooperative dynamic. I have enjoyed this type of interaction with many of my patients, which has enhanced our relationships.

Reliability and follow-through are crucial components in establishing trust over time. Your PCP's clear and timely communication about test results and follow-ups instills confidence in their reliability. Knowing that your provider will inform you promptly about any significant findings or necessary steps enhances your sense of security and trust.

Adhering to prescribed treatments and reporting on outcomes demonstrates your dedication to your health and respect for your PCP's guidance. Consistent record-keeping and sharing of health information further solidify this trust. When you and your PCP have access to accurate and up-to-date health records, it ensures continuity of care and facilitates informed decision-making.

REFLECTION SECTION: STRENGTHENING YOUR RELATIONSHIP WITH YOUR PCP

- **Consistency**: Schedule and attend regular appointments to build a continuous relationship.
- **Honesty**: Be open about your symptoms, lifestyle, and challenges for accurate care.

- **Follow-Through**: Commit to and complete agreed-upon treatment plans.
- **Feedback**: Provide your PCP with feedback on treatments to tailor your care effectively.
- **Empathy**: Show genuine concern and acknowledge each other's perspectives.
- **Reliability**: Ensure clear communication and follow-through on both sides.

Focusing on these strategies can help cultivate a trusting and productive relationship with your primary care provider. This trust enhances your satisfaction with care and leads to better health outcomes, making your healthcare journey more effective and fulfilling.

EFFECTIVE COMMUNICATION: ASKING THE RIGHT QUESTIONS

Preparing for a medical appointment can feel overwhelming, but a little preparation goes a long way—list symptoms and concerns before walking into the doctor's office. Note down any new symptoms, changes in existing conditions, or specific worries you have. This list will help you stay focused during the conversation and ensure you don't forget to mention anything important.

Prioritize Your Questions

Prioritize your questions based on urgency and relevance. If your time with the doctor is limited, having a prioritized list ensures the most critical issues are addressed first. Bring all relevant medical records, including test results, previous diagnoses, and current medications. This gives your healthcare provider a comprehensive understanding of your health history, which is necessary for accurate diagnosis and effective treatment planning.

Knowing what questions to ask can make your medical appointments more productive. Specific questions can guide the conversation and provide the information you need to make informed decisions about your health. For example, ask your healthcare provider, "What are the possible causes of my symptoms?" This question opens the door for a thorough diagnostic discussion. Understanding the potential causes helps you grasp the complexity of your condition and the rationale behind specific tests or treatments.

Inquire, "What are the benefits and risks of the proposed treatment?" Knowing the pros and cons allows you to weigh your options carefully. Each treatment comes with its benefits and potential side effects, and understanding these helps you make choices that align with your health goals and personal preferences. Also, don't hesitate to ask, "Are alternative treatment options available?" Sometimes, there might be different ways to approach your condition, and having options empowers you to choose the one that best fits your lifestyle and comfort level.

Clarifying medical information is necessary to fully understanding your diagnosis and treatment plan. Medical jargon can be confusing, so don't hesitate to ask your provider to explain terms in layman's language.

Importance of Written and Verbal Information

Request written materials or resources for further reading if the information is complex. Having something to refer to later can help solidify your understanding and provide a resource for any follow-up questions. Ask specific questions to clarify medical instructions or follow-up care. Ask for detailed explanations if you're unsure how to take a new medication or what symptoms warrant a follow-up visit. This ensures you're fully informed and can adhere to your treatment plan correctly.

Effective communication during appointments involves speaking clearly and concisely about your symptoms and concerns. Use straightforward language to describe what you're experiencing. For instance, instead of saying, "I don't feel right," specify, "I've had sharp pain in my lower abdomen for the past three days." This specificity helps your provider make an accurate diagnosis. Use "I" statements to express your feelings and preferences, such as, "I feel anxious about starting this new medication because of the potential side effects." This approach personalizes your concerns, helping your provider understand your perspective.

Verify your understanding by summarizing what the provider has explained. Repeat back the key points in your own words. For example, "So, if I understand correctly, I need to take this medication twice a day and come back for a follow-up in two weeks." This recap ensures you and your provider are on the same page. Ask for a recap of the visit at the end of the appointment. This can briefly summarize the key points discussed, the action plan, and any follow-up steps. It reinforces your understanding and provides a clear roadmap for your next steps.

REFLECTION SECTION: PREPARING FOR YOUR NEXT APPOINTMENT

- **Make a List:** List symptoms and concerns before the appointment to stay focused.
- **Prioritize Questions:** List questions in order of importance to ensure critical issues are addressed.

- **Bring Records:** Include medical records, test results, and a list of medications for comprehensive care.
- **Ask Specific Questions:** "What are the possible causes of my symptoms?" "What are the benefits and risks of the proposed treatment?" "Are there alternative treatment options available?"
- **Clarify Information:** Request explanations in layperson's terms, written materials, and precise medical instructions.
- **Effective Communication:** Speak clearly, use "I" statements, verify understanding, and ask for a recap at the end of the visit.

COLLABORATIVE CARE: WORKING WITH SPECIALISTS

Collaborative care is a model designed to address the complexities of managing multiple health conditions by ensuring seamless communication and coordination among various healthcare providers. This approach brings specialists, primary care providers (PCPs), and other healthcare professionals to create a comprehensive and holistic treatment plan tailored to each patient's unique needs. The primary benefit of collaborative care lies in its ability to improve patient outcomes through better coordination and communication. By having all providers on the same page, patients receive consistent and well-rounded care, which enhances their overall experience and satisfaction.

Effective collaboration among healthcare providers is necessary for managing complex health conditions. One of the most essential strategies for facilitating this collaboration is the prompt sharing of medical records and test results. When your PCP and specialists have immediate access to your up-to-date medical information, they can make informed decisions without delay.

Scheduling joint consultations or team meetings is another effective strategy.

Despite being challenging, these sessions allow all involved providers to discuss your treatment plan together, ensuring that every aspect of your care is considered and coordinated. A real concentrated effort must be made to get these sessions to manifest because of the time restraints and the provider shortage I have mentioned earlier in this book. Using patient portals is also beneficial, as these platforms enable you to keep all your providers updated with your latest health information. Encouraging open lines of communication, whether through emails or calls, helps maintain a constant flow of information, reducing the risk of miscommunication and ensuring that all providers are aware of any changes in your condition or treatment plan.

Your role as a patient is equally important in facilitating collaborative care. Keeping all your providers informed about the treatments and medications you are receiving is essential. This means updating your PCP about any new prescriptions or changes in treatment suggested by specialists. Attending follow-up appointments and providing updates on your progress ensures that all your healthcare providers know how you are responding to treatments. Asking for copies of medical reports to share with all your providers helps keep everyone in the loop. Advocacy is also necessary; ensure each provider addresses all your concerns. If you feel something is being overlooked, don't hesitate to bring it up. Your proactive involvement can significantly impact the effectiveness of your care.

Collaborative Care Models

Numerous successful collaborative care models highlight the benefits of this approach. Consider the case of a patient with multiple chronic conditions, such as diabetes and hypertension. Through coordinated care, the patient's PCP, endocrinologist, and cardiologist work together to create a cohesive treatment plan. Regular joint consultations ensure that all aspects of the patient's health are monitored and managed effectively, improving control of both conditions and significantly reducing complications.

Another example involves the successful management of a complex surgical case. A patient requiring multi-stage surgery involving various specialists benefited from a collaborative approach. Surgeons, anesthesiologists, and post-operative care teams held regular meetings to discuss the patient's progress and adjust the treatment plan. This comprehensive coordination minimized risks and enhanced recovery outcomes.

Additionally, integrated mental health and primary care for a patient with depression and diabetes showcase the strength of collaborative care. By integrating behavioral health specialists into the primary care setting, patients receive consistent support for both physical and mental health needs. This integration resulted in improved management of diabetes symptoms and significant improvements in mental well-being.

These examples underscore the importance of a coordinated approach to healthcare, where effective communication and patient involvement play crucial roles. Collaborative care improves health outcomes and enhances the overall patient experience by ensuring that all healthcare providers work together toward a common goal. As we continue to explore the intricacies of navigating the managed care system, understanding the value of collaborative care and how to facilitate it can empower you to take control of your health and achieve better outcomes.

ENDING: SUMMARIZING THE MAIN POINTS

Enhancing your relationship with healthcare providers through trust, effective communication, and collaborative care can significantly improve your health outcomes. As we move forward, let's explore practical steps for navigating the managed care system and making informed decisions about your healthcare.

12

NAVIGATING HEALTHCARE BUREAUCRACY

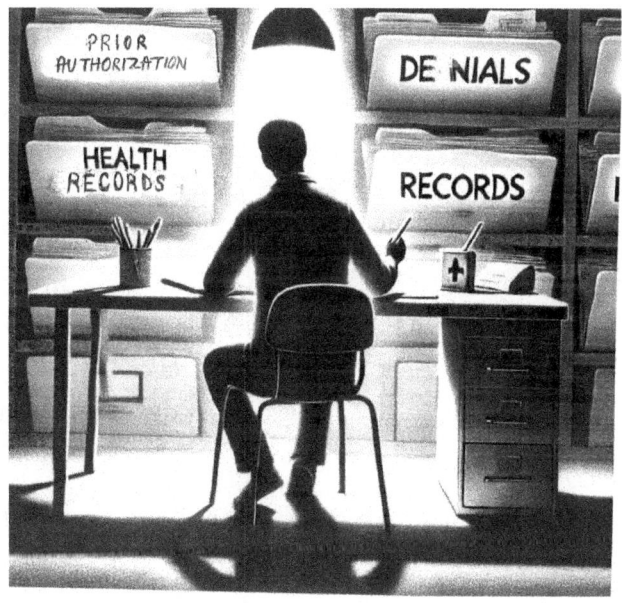

One busy morning, some weeks after my hospitalization owing to a blood clot induced by COVID-19 infection, I opened my mailbox to find it filled with a pile of letters, each more daunting than the last. These consisted of an insurance claim form, a thick packet of explanation of benefits (EOB) statements, and several medical bills. This overwhelming deluge of paperwork is a common experience for many, so healthcare documents must be understood and managed effectively. I'm a doctor and know healthcare paperwork as well as anyone, but this pile of paperwork made me anxious.

MANAGING HEALTHCARE PAPERWORK

Sorting through the stacks of paperwork you're confronted with in healthcare is daunting. Insurance claim forms are typically the first hurdle. They request specific information about your medical care, including dates, provider details, and services provided. Filling these out correctly is essential so your insurance will pay for the services. Delays or denials will result from incomplete or incorrect information, adding to an already stressful process.

Explanation of Benefits

Explanation of benefits (EOB) statements are also an important document. They detail what your insurance has paid, what you owe, and what was rejected. They itemize the cost of each service, indicating what was paid by insurance and what remains your charge.

On the other hand, medical bills and invoices come directly from healthcare providers, and the services' fees are itemized. They may be confusing, citing numerous codes and jargon that are not clearly understood. You need to reconcile your EOB (Explanation of Benefits) with your medical bills to ensure accuracy and prevent overcharging.

Most medical treatments and procedures require authorization and consent forms. These outline the benefits and risks of a procedure so that you are informed and can consent to the treatment you will receive. They document that you have been informed about what will take place and have consented to the procedure.

Developing a Filing System

It is essential to keep all of these documents organized.

A filing system with labeled files for different categories of documents can make everything accessible. For example, you may have separate files for insurance claim forms, EOB statements, medical bills, and consent forms. Electronic aids and software programs to scan and store electronic versions can also prove helpful. They enable you to keep electronic copies of all your documents, which are readily available and can be transmitted to healthcare professionals when required.

Another helpful technique is keeping a chronological list of medical appointments and treatments. This list will enable you to track your medical progress, making it easier to refer back to previous treatments and recall your medical history. Having reminders for insurance claims and bill payments will help you avoid forgetting critical deadlines, allowing you to stay on top of your financial responsibilities and avoid incurring late fees.

It is just as important to understand and review your healthcare records as it is to keep them organized. Reading your EOBs and medical bills carefully will help you identify errors and prevent confusion. Look for common sections in these forms, such as service dates, provider names, and service descriptions. Compare these pieces of information with your insurance coverage to verify that they all match. Verifying charges and services rendered safeguards you against payment for services never received or those charged by mistake.

SETTLING DISAGREEMENTS

If you identify mistakes or disagreements, it is essential to resolve them promptly. To do so, contact your healthcare provider's billing department for clarification. They are often in a position to explain charges and correct errors. Submitting written dispute letters to your insurance company is also an effective way to resolve issues. State the discrepancy clearly, include any supporting documents, and ask for review. Record every correspondence and decision, as having a clear record of your dispute's progression and a well-documented paper trail is crucial.

At times, it can be challenging to negotiate conflicts independently, and seeking the aid of patient advocacy organizations can be helpful. These organizations specialize in navigating healthcare bureaucracy and can offer valuable insights and guidance. They can help you understand your rights, communicate effectively with healthcare providers and insurers, and negotiate to resolve disputes.

CHECKLIST: ORGANIZING AND MANAGING HEALTHCARE PAPERWORK

- **Create a Filing System**
    - Label folders for insurance claim forms, EOB statements, medical bills, and consent forms.
    - Group documents by type for easy access.
- **Utilize Digital Tools**
    - Scan and save electronic versions of all documents.

- Utilize apps for organization and quick access.
- **Keep a Chronological Record**
  - Maintain a complete record of medical appointments and treatments in chronological order.
  - Record dates, providers, and services performed.
- **Create Reminders**
  - Set reminders for bill due dates and insurance claims.
  - Monitor critical deadlines to prevent late fees.
- **Read and Comprehend Documents**
  - Read medical bills and EOBs thoroughly.
  - Compare information with insurance coverage.
- **Resolve Discrepancies**
  - Call billing departments for clarification.
  - Send formal dispute letters to insurance providers.
  - Document all communication and resolutions.
- **Seek Assistance**
  - Contact patient advocacy groups for help.
  - Leverage their experience in dealing with healthcare bureaucracy.

Using these methods, you can navigate the generally overwhelming world of healthcare documents with greater ease and confidence, stay in control and organized, and manage your healthcare experience effectively.

COMPREHENDING AND ORGANIZING YOUR HEALTH RECORDS

Organizing your health records is important to assuming control of your healthcare. Numerous health records are available that you should be aware of. Personal Health Records (PHRs) are sets of your medical records. They can contain your medical history, diagnosis, medications, immunizations, and other relevant information. They provide an overview of your health, allowing you and your healthcare providers to conveniently access your health information.

On the other hand, electronic health records (EHRs) are electronic forms of the paper charts kept by healthcare providers. These records are exchanged between various healthcare settings to make your health history accessible to all your providers. These contain detailed information like test results, imaging reports, and treatment plans, which are vital for coordinated care. Test results and imaging reports are essential parts of your health records.

They offer detailed information about your medical condition and direct your treatment plans. These records contain the results of blood tests, X-rays, MRIs, and other diagnostic tests that enable your healthcare providers to make informed decisions about your health. Immunization records are also a vital part of your health records. These records track all your vaccinations and keep you up to date with your immunizations, protecting you from many diseases.

Requesting Copies of Health Records

Requesting copies of health records is a simple yet tedious task to obtain and receive copies of your health records. First, call your healthcare provider's medical records department. You will need to complete and return a release form, provide the necessary records, and specify the purpose for which you are requesting the records. It is advantageous to familiarize yourself with the process and timeline for accessing records, as it may take anywhere from a few days to a few weeks, depending on the provider. Know your Health Insurance Portability and Accountability Act (HIPAA) rights. HIPAA provides you the right to access your health information and provides confidentiality of your records. Learn about these rights to obtain and manage your health records effectively.

Maintaining Accurate, Up-to-Date Personal Health Records

An updated personal health record has several advantages. Keeping records of your treatments and medical history helps provide new healthcare professionals with accurate details, enabling continuity of care. This is crucial if you have long-term conditions, as it enables you to track your treatment progress and make informed decisions about your care. Having immediate access to health information also prepares you for emergencies. In emergencies, having your health records with you can enable healthcare professionals to make quick and informed decisions regarding your care. Keeping your health records organized and readily available for proper management is necessary.

Digital patient portals and apps are incredibly convenient for this purpose. They enable you to electronically store and view your health records, making it convenient to update and share them with your healthcare professionals. An electronic storage system in one location ensures that all your health data is readily available, with a reduced risk of losing vital documents. Regularly updating your files with new information, such as recent test results or updated medication schedules, ensures that your health records are current. Sharing pertinent records with all your healthcare providers who manage your care guarantees integrated and holistic care.

TIPS FOR MANAGING HEALTH RECORDS

- **Utilize Digital Patient Portals and Health Apps**
    - Electronically store and retrieve your health records.

- Add new information to update records.
- Share records with clinicians.
- **Create a Centralized Digital Storage System**
  - Keep all your health data in one place.
  - Reduce the risk of losing important documents.
- **Regularly Update Records**
  - Add recent test results and medication changes.
  - Ensure that records are up to date at all times.
- **Share Relevant Records**
  - Promote coordinated and comprehensive care.
  - Give complete and current information to all your healthcare providers.

By organizing your health records, you can actively participate in your healthcare, ensuring that you and your providers have current and accurate information. This enhances the quality of your care, enabling you to make informed decisions about your health.

UNDERSTANDING THE REFERRAL PROCESS

Although the managed care system's referral process may be complicated, understanding how it works can significantly improve your healthcare experience.

The gatekeepers in this system are the primary care providers (PCPs), who provide you with the care you require and keep costs in line. Should specialized care be necessary, your primary care physician (PCP) will assess your situation and, if required, refer you to a specialist. This is a prerequisite as most policies require a referral to reimburse specialist visits. If not, you could face massive out-of-pocket expenses. Getting a referral is a stepwise process.

You will need to schedule an appointment with your primary care physician (PCP) first to discuss your symptoms and concerns. Your primary care physician (PCP) will decide during the visit whether you should receive a referral to a specialist. If they do, they'll give you a referral form or forward it to the specialist. It's a good idea to know your insurance needs for referrals. Your plan might have limitations on which specialists you must see and which services need referrals. Clarifying these points with your insurance company saves time and prevents additional charges. Early communication is the most effective way of getting timely and proper referrals.

Begin by making an appointment with your PCP to discuss your referral needs. After you've been referred, confirm arrangements with your specialist and PCP. Doing this guarantees that everyone knows what's taking place and your appointment is scheduled in the correct location. Following up with the insurance company to confirm referral approval and to confirm that the insurance company has all it needs from the PCP is also important. Such a confirmation can avert any interruption in your care. Also, inquire about referral expiration dates and necessary renewals so there is no gap in your care. Typical problems in the referral process are delays in approval and processing, communication breakdown between specialists, PCPs, and insurance providers, and the unavailability of specialists in the network.

Delays can happen if the forms are not completed or if there is a backlog at the insurance company. To avoid this, make sure all forms are completed properly and follow up every now and then with your PCP and insurance provider. Miscommunication can be resolved through open and honest communication with everyone involved. If there are not enough specialists in your network, you might have to request out-of-network care. This request contains a valid explanation of the need for an out-of-network specialist, along with supporting documentation from your medical providers.

PATIENT INVOLVEMENT IN THE PROCESS

Patient involvement in the referral process is critical. Remaining active and involved can greatly contribute to the quality and effectiveness of your care. Begin by seeking complete information about the referral and specialist care. Knowing why you are being referred and what you can expect from the specialist can prepare you. Organize all pertinent health records before seeing the specialist, such as past test results and treatment strategies. This preparation ensures the specialist has all the information required to provide the best care possible.

Effective communication with your PCP and specialist is necessary. Express your symptoms, concerns, and expectations clearly. This helps both providers understand your needs and coordinate your care accordingly. The second most important aspect is following up and coordination between providers. Inform your PCP about the outcome and new treatment plans once you have visited your specialist. This notification helps your PCP incorporate the specialist's advice into your general care plan, providing continuity and holistic care.

SUMMARY OF THE REFERRAL PROCESS

As I completed this section in my book, I wanted to stress to readers how vital it is to know how to work through prior authorizations. Even though I no longer have my medical clinic, I still advise my family and friends on how to do so because it is challenging.

One wrong move or pause can easily deny your prior authorization. Thus, in conclusion, navigating the referral process within managed care networks involves knowing the role of PCPs, adhering to the process of getting referrals, and playing an active role in solving possible problems. By playing an active role and communicating effectively with everyone involved, you can get the specialist care you need in an effective and efficient manner.

13

ADDRESSING MENTAL HEALTH IN MANAGED CARE

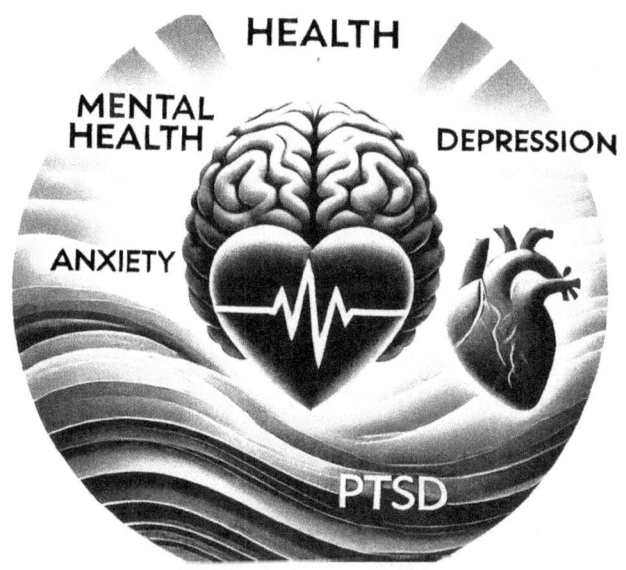

Laura had come to see me on a particularly slow day at the office. I learned later that she was a young executive who had carried an enormous emotional burden in silence. As she sat in my office, her hands shaking, she spoke about how sadness and fatigue had overtaken her life. She had a destructive marriage, three children, and fear of leaving. She shared that she has now become more anxious and is starting to have panic attacks. Her glowing, confident exterior masked the struggle she had with every day going into her house. Laura's story is unfortunately not unique because mental health struggles affect many; however, such struggles often get hidden due to stigma or even lack of awareness.

Addressing mental health needs within MCS is paramount because, without it, a true healthcare system that supports all aspects of health for any given individual cannot be created.

MEETING MENTAL HEALTH NEEDS

Mental health diagnoses can range from conditions that are extremely serious to ones less debilitating. The following are some of the more common conditions that are initially diagnosed by a Primary Care Physician.

- **Depression:** Feelings of pervasive sadness, loss of interest in activities, overwhelming fatigue. Simple things, such as getting out of bed or mingling with other people, become impossible tasks.
- **Anxiety Disorders:** Groundless fears, excessive and irrational; panic attacks and symptoms like muscular tension or tightness in the chest make it difficult to deal with everyday challenges.
- **Bipolar Disorder:** Characterized by extreme mood swings, when depressive episodes, profound sadness, and lethargy follow manic episodes, high energy, euphoria, and impulsiveness.
- **Post-Traumatic Stress Disorder (PTSD):** This is a trauma-inflicted disorder characterized by flashbacks, high levels of arousal, and avoidance behaviors.

- **ADHD**: Typically shows patterns of inattentiveness, hyperactivity, lack of focus, and impulsivity, usually beginning in childhood

Why Early Detection Is Important

The earlier such conditions are caught, the better the outcomes. Early intervention keeps symptoms from increasing to crisis points, improves the quality of life, and diminishes the chance of complications involving substance abuse or self-harm. The sooner mental health difficulties are picked up, the timelier and more successful the treatments in ensuring emotional stability and functional well-being can be.

How to Recognize Mental Health Issues

Be self-aware. Keeping a mental health journal to track moods, symptoms, and triggers can reveal patterns that provide insight. Online screening tools, such as those available through the National Institute of Mental Health, can help identify the need for professional treatment. Behavioral changes, such as withdrawal from friends, disrupted sleep, or changes in appetite, are potent warning signs. Friends or family members may also have valuable feedback as they notice changes in someone's demeanor.

OVERCOMING STIGMA

Stigma is perhaps the major deterrent to treatment, silencing so many in their suffering. The time has come to break the silence.

- **Educate Yourself and Others:** Mental health conditions are not moral weaknesses but illnesses. Realizing this can minimize stigma.

- **Talk About It Openly:** Sharing experiences normalizes the conversations about mental health, and others will find it easier to seek help.
- **Find Support Groups:** Being part of communities where you can share your story without judgment helps cultivate acceptance and understanding.
- **Advocate for Awareness:** Supporting mental health education in your community can encourage more people to prioritize their mental well-being.

HOW TO ACCESS MENTAL HEALTH SERVICES IN A MANAGED CARE

Mental health services in MCS can be confusing, but the knowledge of options certainly helps.

- **Outpatient Therapy and Counseling**: Regular sessions with a licensed therapist offer a safe space to deal with mental health concerns. Cognitive-behavioral treatment or talk therapy is offered according to the individual's needs.
- **Psychiatric Evaluations and Medication Management**: The psychiatrist will consider conditions and prescription medication, adjusting dosages to better manage symptoms. It may take some time to find just the right medication and dosage, but it is often necessary to achieve stability.
- **Intensive Outpatient Programs (IOPs) and Partial Hospitalization Programs (PHPs)**: For those needing more structured care, IOPs offer multiple therapy sessions a week while the patient can still go about their daily life. PHPs are more intensive, offering full-day therapy sessions to address severe mental health challenges.
- **Crisis Intervention Services**: Hotlines, mobile crisis

units, and walk-in centers offer immediate support and stabilization for acute crises.

NAVIGATING INSURANCE COVERAGE FOR MENTAL HEALTH

Know your insurance benefits, which is important in accessing care:

- **Review Your Plan:** Look at what mental health services are covered, including copays and deductibles.
- **Identify In-Network Providers:** Using therapists or psychiatrists in your network reduces costs significantly.
- **Obtain Authorizations:** Specialized services like IOPs or PHPs may require prior authorization from your insurer. Have your healthcare provider submit the necessary documentation to avoid delays.

Your primary care provider (PCP) can also play a key role in navigating coverage. During routine check-ups, PCPs can screen for mental health concerns and provide referrals to specialists, along with prior authorization if needed. Their collaboration with mental health providers ensures integrated care that addresses physical and emotional needs.

ALTERNATIVE RESOURCES FOR MENTAL HEALTH CARE

If traditional routes feel out of reach, consider these options:

- **Community Mental Health Centers:** Offer services on a sliding scale fee based on income. Usually located in your town.

- **Nonprofit Organizations:** Many provide free or low-cost counseling.
- **National Alliance on Mental Illness (NAMI):** NAMI is the largest grassroots mental health organization in the US, offering advocacy, education, support, and public awareness to improve the lives of those affected by mental illness. They have over 700 state organizations and affiliates nationwide. Visit their website at NAMI.org.
- **Active Minds:** Targeting young adults ages fourteen to twenty-five, Active Minds aims to raise mental health awareness and promote education via peer interaction. Its mission is to decrease stigma and increase help-seeking behaviors. They have a crisis text line and phone number: 1-800-273-talk (8255). Visit their website at activeminds.org.
- **Fountain House:** This organization advocates for people with serious mental illness by offering community involvement, housing, employment, and educational resources. Fountain House developed the Clubhouse Model of Psychosocial Rehabilitation.
- **Crisis Text Line:** Provides free, twenty-four-seven confidential support via text. Crisis Text Line connects people in crisis with trained crisis counselors. To contact them, text HOME to 741741.
- **Online Therapy Platforms:** Telehealth services offer convenience, allowing users to connect with licensed therapists and doctors from the comfort of their own homes.
- **Employee Assistance Programs:** Often underutilized, EAPs provide employees with free, confidential counseling to address a range of personal and work-related issues.

INTEGRATING MENTAL AND PHYSICAL HEALTH CARE

Our mental and physical health are deeply connected. Remember Robert, the middle-aged man with diabetes and depression. He was taking his medications as prescribed, but his blood sugar levels remained unpredictable. It wasn't until we started treating his depression, in addition to his diabetes, that his health began to improve. Robert's experience illustrates the need to treat the whole person, not just isolated symptoms.

The Benefits of Integration

- Good mental health facilitates the management of chronic physical conditions, such as diabetes or heart disease.
- Care coordination avoids redundant tests, unnecessary treatments, and hospitalizations, saving time, money, and stress.
- Patients feel better cared for, leading to higher satisfaction and better outcomes.

STRATEGIES FOR INTEGRATED CARE

Integration requires collaboration. Collaborative care models integrate primary care physicians (PCPs), mental health professionals, and specialists in the development of tailored care plans. Shared EHRs facilitate effective communication among providers, ensuring that all parties are on the same page. Regular team meetings regarding patient progress keep care dynamic and responsive.

A patient's active role in their treatment, joint setting of objectives, and raising awareness about the interconnection between mental and physical health problems will help them manage the conditions independently.

REAL-LIFE SUCCESS STORY: JANICE

I had a patient, Janice, who had diabetes and depression, and she could manage neither. Of course, her depression indeed worsened when her diabetes was uncontrolled and vice versa. Through a coordinated care system between her therapist and me, she got her blood sugar in better control and got relief from depression. That holistic approach transformed her life, proving that integrated care is effective.

CONCLUSION: WHOLE-PERSON HEALTH

Addressing mental health in managed care is about combining mental and physical health together to treat the whole person. By seeking collaborative care models, reducing stigma, and utilizing available resources, we can ultimately develop a system that supports mental well-being as an integral part of overall health.

Realistically, an obstacle to the advancement of this model is the reduction of doctors in all specialties after the pandemic. However, this is not an excuse to underutilize the resourcese that are available.

In the next chapter, I'll discuss patient rights and advocacy. I will also help you understand how to navigate the healthcare system and take charge of your care.

14

LEGAL RIGHTS AND PATIENT ADVOCACY

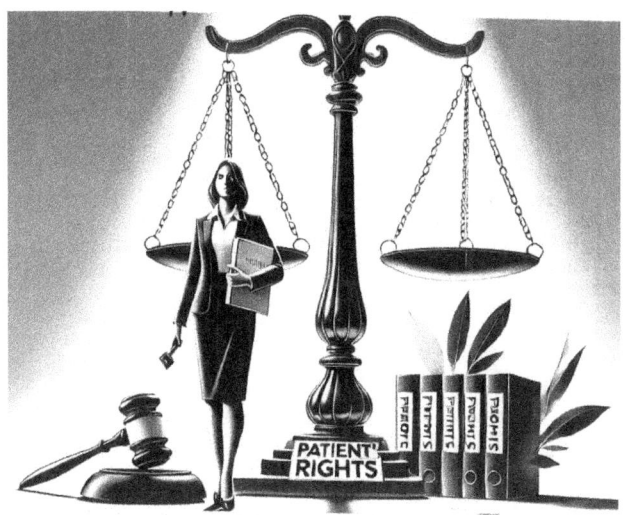

In my thirty-eight years of practicing medicine, I have spoken to many patients who were confused about the surgeries they had been recommended to have. I have observed this in many instances and have seen numerous scenarios where patients are apprehensive about advocating for themselves. Some patients, without further inquiry, just won't have the surgery. Some seem fearful of inquiring more about the surgery, fearing that this may offend the surgeon.

I remember a patient, Margaret, who was particularly distressed and verbose about her concerns. She faced a difficult decision: She had been undergoing treatment for a chronic condition and was now being asked to consider a surgical procedure. Margaret sounded overwhelmed by the medical jargon and the endless stack of consent forms. "How do I know I'm making the right choice?" she asked. Her concerns were valid, but she was hesitant to voice them to the surgeon. Like many patients, Margaret must understand her rights to make an informed decision.

This chapter helps you understand your legal rights as a patient, equipping you with the tools and confidence to navigate the healthcare system effectively.

THE RIGHT TO INFORMED CONSENT

One of our most critical rights as patients is the right to informed consent. Before you undergo any medical procedure, your healthcare provider must explain:

- The treatment options available
- The risks and benefits of each option
- Any alternatives to the procedure
- What could happen if you choose to do nothing

This information must be presented in a manner that is easy to understand. Your healthcare provider's job is to ensure you're comfortable and have all your questions answered before you sign anything. Beyond a formality, written consent is your assurance that you're making a well-informed decision.

THE RIGHT TO ACCESS YOUR MEDICAL RECORDS

Your medical records are more than just charts and notes—they're a key part of managing your health. You have the right to access and obtain copies of your records, whether for a second opinion, switching providers, or keeping a personal health history.

To request your records:

1. Contact the medical records department of your healthcare provider or hospital.
2. Complete a request form and provide the required identification.
3. Be aware of potential processing fees and the standard thirty-day timeframe for receiving your records.

Review your records for accuracy. If you spot an error, you have the right to request corrections. Maintaining up-to-date records is crucial for ensuring the continuity of care and ensuring that your treatment plan aligns with your specific needs.

THE RIGHT TO PRIVACY AND CONFIDENTIALITY

The Health Insurance Portability and Accountability Act (HIPPA) protects your personal health information. HIPAA ensures that your medical records and personal details remain confidential unless you authorize their release.

Healthcare providers, insurance companies, and other covered entities are required to:

- Provide you with a written notice of their privacy practices

- Use only the minimum necessary information for any purpose

If you believe your privacy rights have been violated, you can file a complaint with the US Department of Health and Human Services (HHS). Knowing this right can give you peace of mind when sharing sensitive health information.

THE RIGHT TO REFUSE TREATMENT

You also have the right to refuse treatment—even if your healthcare provider believes it's in your best interest. This decision should be based on a thorough understanding of the risks and consequences, which your provider must clearly explain.

For example, patients often exercise this right when considering invasive procedures or treatments with significant risks. You need to be empowered to ask detailed questions about your procedure. If you decline treatment, your provider should respect your choice without pressuring you. Your decision and reasoning should be documented in your medical record.

REFLECTION SECTION: KNOW YOUR RIGHTS

- **Right to Informed Consent**: Ensure your healthcare provider explains all treatment options, risks, and benefits in understandable terms. Ask questions until you feel confident in your understanding before providing written consent.
- **Right to Access Medical Records:** Contact your healthcare provider's medical records department to request copies of your records. Verify their accuracy and request corrections if needed.

- **Right to Privacy and Confidentiality**: Familiarize yourself with HIPAA regulations and your healthcare provider's privacy practices. Report any violations to the US Department of Health and Human Services.
- **Right to Refuse Treatment:** You have the right to decline any medical intervention. Make informed decisions by discussing the implications with your healthcare provider.

PERSONAL STORY

A story close to my heart is the horrific medical error that injured my now ninety-two-year-old friend Jenna. Jenna worked as an assistant in a medical office, handling payroll and clerical work. She was active and working before her injury.

A shoe was on the floor in her bedroom, and she tripped and fell. She broke her right hip, which is a horrible ordeal for anyone, but especially a ninety-year-old. I found out about the broken hip when she was hospitalized and sent for surgery. I assumed she was getting a total hip replacement, but instead, unbeknownst to me at the time, the surgeon placed a rod into a ninety-year-old femur without cement augmentation. She had complications because of the softness of her bones.

Within a month later, she had to go back into surgery and have the rod removed. Jenna then got a total hip replacement. Putting a rod into her femur was less costly, less complicated, and safer. Still, it may not be the correct surgery for an osteoporotic ninety-year-old without cement augmentation of her bone. I believe the surgeon's decision-making might have been flawed. I think more questions should have been asked. I was distraught because her family, who I knew, did not inform me earlier so I could have been involved with talking to the surgeon. I would have questioned his decision to place a rod in a ninety-two-year-old femur that had severe osteoporosis. I'm not sure if I was right, but at least the question would have been asked.

Our conversation might not have changed anything, but it would have clarified his decision. Jenna has problems with pain during weight bearing of her right thigh still two years later. She had two major surgeries on the same extremity within a month, which I believe is at least partially responsible for the excess pain and difficulty walking she experiences today. Otherwise, Jenna is a healthy ninety-two-year-old but is mainly limited to her room because of severe pain and difficulty walking. I discovered that detailed information about each surgery was not requested and not provided, so an informed choice could not have been made, which could be considered a breach of care.

LEGAL RECOURSE IN CASES OF MEDICAL NEGLIGENCE

Medical negligence occurs when a healthcare provider fails to meet the accepted standard of care, resulting in harm.

Duty of Care: The provider must have had a professional responsibility to care for you.

1. **Breach of Care**: The provider failed to act in a manner consistent with the standards of a competent professional.
2. **Causation**: The breach directly caused you harm.
3. **Damages**: You suffered injury, emotional distress, or financial loss.

FILING A MEDICAL MALPRACTICE CLAIM

If you believe you've been a victim of medical negligence, take these steps:

1. **Consult a medical malpractice attorney.** Look for an attorney experienced in similar cases. They can guide you through the legal process and explain your options.
2. **Gather evidence.** Collect medical records, photographs, witness statements, and expert opinions.
3. **File a complaint.** Your attorney will help you file a complaint within the statute of limitations, typically one to three years from the date of the incident or its discovery.

The outcomes of malpractice cases vary. While most are resolved through financial settlements to cover medical bills, lost wages, and pain and suffering, others may involve formal apologies or corrective actions.

UTILIZING PATIENT ADVOCACY SERVICES

Navigating the healthcare system can be overwhelming, especially during stressful situations. Patient advocacy services are invaluable for providing clarity and support. Also, using a trusted friend or relative can be an outstanding advocate.

What Can Patient Advocates Do?

- **Explain Diagnoses and Treatment Options**: They simplify medical jargon and ensure you understand your condition and care plan.
- **Attend Appointments**: Advocates can ask questions, take notes, and ensure nothing is overlooked.

- **Resolve Billing and Insurance Issues**: They can help you understand your bills, negotiate with insurance companies, and secure the benefits you're entitled to.

Finding the Right Advocate

To find a qualified advocate:

1. **Research Organizations**: Look into local and national patient advocacy groups.
2. **Verify Credentials: Ensure they possess the necessary** expertise to meet your specific needs.
3. **Ask for Recommendations**: Consider consulting with healthcare providers or support groups for trusted referrals.
4. **Understand Costs**: Some advocates charge flat fees or hourly rates, so clarify these details upfront.

The Benefits of Patient Advocacy

Having a patient advocate by your side can:

- Improve communication with your healthcare team.
- Increase your confidence and understanding of complex medical issues.
- Reduce stress during hospital stays and treatments.
- Ensure that your care aligns with your values and needs.

For example, a patient advocate might help you coordinate care for a complex surgical procedure, ensure you understand a serious diagnosis, or resolve disputes with your insurance company.

CONCLUSION

Understanding your legal rights and knowing how to advocate for yourself effectively is crucial for navigating the healthcare system. From exercising your right to informed consent to seeking support through patient advocacy, these tools empower you to take control of your care.

As we move forward, the next chapter will examine how the managed care system tailors services for special populations, highlighting strategies to meet the diverse healthcare needs of these populations.

Note: Near the end of the book, a list of advocacy organizations is provided for contact if needed.

15

SPECIAL POPULATIONS AND MANAGED CARE

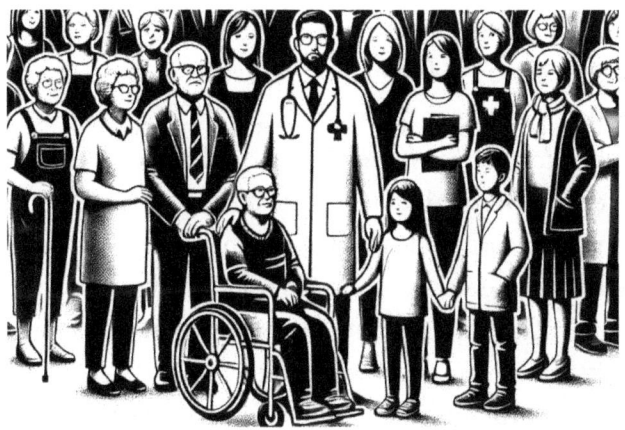

Navigating the managed care system (MCS) can be challenging. Still, the journey can be particularly complex for special populations like seniors, children, and individuals with chronic illnesses or disabilities. These groups often have unique healthcare needs that require extra attention and tailored strategies. This chapter will examine how the MCS addresses these needs and how individuals and families can maximize the use of available resources.

SENIORS IN MANAGED CARE: TACKLING THE CHALLENGES

One of my most memorable patients, Mrs. Thompson, was an eighty-two-year-old woman who came to my office with a bag full of medications and a look of confusion. Like many seniors, she was managing multiple chronic conditions—hypertension, diabetes, and arthritis—and struggling to keep track of everything. Her story perfectly exemplifies the unique needs of older adults in managed care.

Common Healthcare Needs for Seniors

- **Managing Chronic Conditions**: Seniors often require close monitoring and treatment adjustments for conditions such as high blood pressure, diabetes, and arthritis. If left unchecked, these conditions can lead to severe complications, such as heart failure or mobility loss.
- **Preventive Screenings**: Routine tests, such as mammograms, colonoscopies, and bone density scans, are vital for early detection of issues like cancer or osteoporosis. Catching these problems early can mean less invasive treatments and better outcomes.
- **Mental Health Support**: Depression and dementia are common among seniors, often exacerbated by isolation or chronic illness. Specialized care plans can help maintain mental well-being and manage symptoms. One of my favorite activities as a doctor is when I owned a company where I hired LCSWs to help me provide mental health group sessions to nursing home patients

The Role of Medicare

Medicare plays a central role in senior healthcare within the MCS. It's essential to understand the options:

- **Original Medicare**: Includes Part A (hospital care) and Part B (doctor visits). You can add Part D for prescription drugs. Think of it as a buffet—you pick what you need.
- **Medicare Advantage**: A bundled plan managed by private insurers that combines Parts A, B, and often Part D, plus additional benefits such as dental and vision care.
- **Supplemental Plans:** These include plans like Medigap, which can help cover out-of-pocket costs, while Medicare eligibility typically begins at age sixty-five. Understanding enrollment windows is critical to avoid penalties or coverage gaps.

Choosing the Right Plan

When selecting a managed care plan (Medicare Advantage), seniors should:

- Compare costs, coverage, and provider networks.
- Evaluate specific needs, such as prescription drug coverage or access to specialists.
- Check for additional benefits, such as dental, vision, or fitness programs.
- Use resources like State Health Insurance Assistance Programs (SHIPs) for free counseling.

PEDIATRIC CARE IN THE MANAGED CARE SYSTEM

Children have their own unique healthcare needs, from routine check-ups to managing chronic conditions. Pediatric care within the MCS focuses on prevention, early intervention, and comprehensive management.

Core Components of Pediatric Care

- **Well-Child Visits and Immunizations**: These regular check-ups track growth development, and vaccines are administered to protect against serious illnesses like measles and polio. These are crucial, as evidenced by the increased morbidity and mortality in the recent measles outbreak in the United States.
- **Developmental Screenings**: Assessments for conditions such as autism or speech delays help ensure early intervention, which can lead to improved long-term outcomes.
- **Managing Chronic Conditions**: Common issues like asthma require careful monitoring and medication management. For ADHD, it requires a combination of behavioral therapy, education, and possibly medication..

Nonprofit and Advocacy Organizations for Children

1. **Easterseals:**
   - Their websites provide services such as therapy, inclusive childcare, and support for children with disabilities and their families.
2. **The Arc (thearc.org):**
   - Their website focuses on advocacy, educational programs, and community-based support for

individuals with intellectual and developmental disabilities.
3. **United Cerebral Palsy (UCP):**
    - Their website offers education, therapy, and assistive technology for children with cerebral palsy and other disabilities.
4. **Special Olympics:**
    - Their website promotes sports and fitness opportunities for children and adults with intellectual disabilities.
5. **National Down Syndrome Society (NDSS):**
    - Their website provides resources, advocacy, and educational materials for families of children with Down syndrome.
6. **Autism Speaks:**
    - Their website offers early screening resources, educational support, and advocacy for children with autism spectrum disorders.

Healthcare and Therapy Programs

1. **Shriners Hospitals for Children**
    - Provides orthopedic care, therapy, and rehabilitation services for children with physical disabilities.
2. **Children's Miracle Network Hospitals**
    - Supports families of children with disabilities through healthcare services and community programs.
3. **Early Intervention Programs (EIP)**
    - State-administered programs for children under three with developmental delays or disabilities.

Supporting Nutrition and Activity

Good nutrition and regular physical activity are foundational for healthy development. Pediatricians can help parents create balanced diets and encourage exercise to prevent obesity and related health issues.

Public Health Programs for Children

Programs such as Medicaid and the Children's Health Insurance Program (CHIP) offer affordable coverage to eligible families. These programs ensure access to preventive care, doctor visits, and hospital services. Families can enroll through the Health Insurance Marketplace or state agencies.

Choosing the Right Pediatrician

- Look for board certification and experience in pediatrics.
- Ensure access to specialists, such as allergists or neurologists, within the network.
- Seek recommendations from other parents or community resources.

MANAGING CHRONIC ILLNESSES AND DISABILITIES

For individuals managing chronic conditions or disabilities, navigating the MCS can feel like a full-time job. The process can be overwhelming, from coordinating care among specialists to securing necessary equipment.

Challenges Faced

- **Care Coordination**: Managing multiple providers and treatments can lead to conflicting advice or gaps in care. Communication is vital to ensuring everyone is on the same page. Keep a comprehensive health history file using Electronic Health Records shared by providers.
- **Complex Medication Regimens**: Juggling multiple prescriptions with varying schedules can be confusing and risky without proper management tools like pill organizers or apps. Examples are Medisafe, Mango Health, Pill Reminder-Meds Alarm, CareZone, and MyTherapy.
- **Accessing Equipment**: Obtaining wheelchairs, CPAP machines, or orthotics often requires navigating insurance approvals and completing extensive documentation; we discuss this in Chapters 2, 7, and 12.

Strategies for Success

- Establish a medical home with a primary care provider (PCP) who oversees your care and makes referrals as needed.
- Use care coordinators provided by managed care plans to streamline appointments and align treatments.
- Keep detailed records of your medical history, medications, and past treatments to share with new providers.
- Schedule regular follow-ups to monitor progress and adjust treatment plans proactively.

Self-Management and Advocacy

Educating yourself about your condition empowers you to take an active role in your care. Support groups and advocacy organizations can provide emotional support, practical advice, and resources to help you navigate the system. Setting realistic goals and tracking your progress can also help you stay motivated and focused.

Resources for Support

- **Area Agencies on Aging (AAAs)**: Provide meal programs, transportation, and advocacy for seniors.
- **Early Intervention Programs**: Offer therapies for children with developmental delays. **Early Intervention (EI) Services (IDEA Part C)**: A federally mandated program under the Individuals with Disabilities Education Act (IDEA) provides therapy services for children under the age of three. Find your state's Early Head Start program.
- **Nonprofit Organizations**: Groups such as AARP and the National Multiple Sclerosis Society offer educational resources, support groups, and financial assistance. The Arc offers hospital-based programs for children. Check out websites like Boston Children's Hospital and Kennedy Krieger Institute. Look for University-Based Early Intervention Clinics.
- **Government Programs**: Programs like Social Security Disability Insurance (SSDI) help alleviate financial burdens for individuals with disabilities.

REFLECTION SECTION: KEY TAKEAWAYS

- **For Seniors:**
  - Compare Medicare Advantage plans and assess their coverage of prescription drugs and additional benefits.
  - Utilize resources such as AARP and SHIPs for guidance.
- **For Children:**
  - Ensure routine check-ups and immunizations are up to date.
  - Explore public health programs, such as Medicaid or CHIP, for affordable care.
  - Find information about programs for children with disabilities.
- **For Chronic Illnesses and Disabilities:**
  - Establish a medical home with a trusted PCP.
  - Utilize patient advocacy organizations for support and resources. (Advocacy programs are listed on Page 86.)

CONCLUSION

Special populations face unique challenges within the managed care system, but understanding the available resources and strategies can significantly improve their health outcomes. Whether navigating Medicare, ensuring comprehensive pediatric care, or managing chronic conditions, the right tools and support can empower individuals and families to achieve better health outcomes.

In the next chapter, we will examine the systemic challenges of managed care and explore practical solutions for optimizing the system.

16

FUTURE TRENDS IN MANAGED CARE

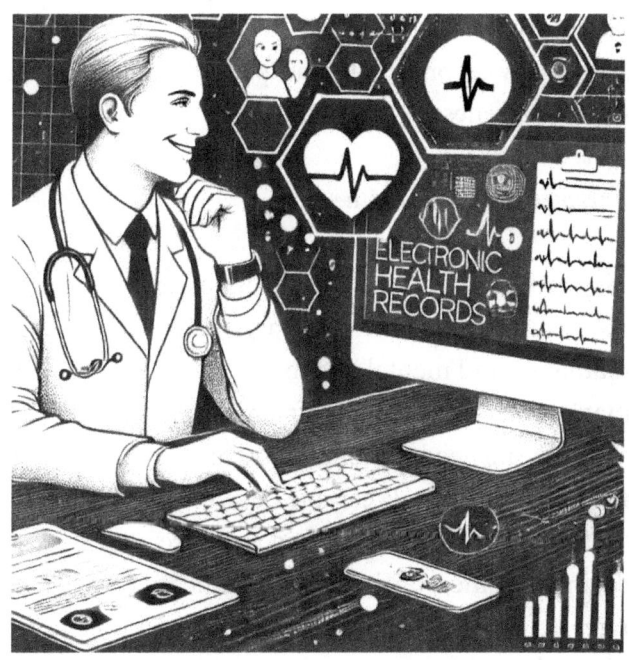

I currently work for a telehealth company. I see patients living in rural areas where many specialists are unavailable. A patient, Maria, informed me during a telemedicine visit she lived in a remote location and struggled with chronic migraines. The nearest neurologist was hours away, making regular visits nearly impossible. Maria finally found a neurologist who utilized telehealth. Maria could consult with her specialist without leaving her home, significantly improving her condition. Of course, she had medical records with previous testing and exams that confirmed her diagnosis of migraines. Maria's experience offers a glimpse into the future of healthcare, where telehealth, digital tools, and innovative care models transform how we deliver and receive care.

THE FUTURE OF TELEHEALTH AND DIGITAL HEALTH

The rise of telehealth has been nothing short of transformative. Before the pandemic, only about 5% of patients used telehealth. Today, that number has surged to over 25 percent, and it continues to grow as providers and patients recognize its convenience and effectiveness.

Key Advancements in Telehealth

1. **Specialized Virtual Care**: Telehealth extends beyond primary care to specialties such as cardiology, dermatology, and mental health. Imagine consulting a dermatologist or cardiologist from your living room, eliminating the need for lengthy travel.
2. **Remote Monitoring**: Wearable devices now track health metrics, such as heart rate, blood pressure, and glucose levels, in real time, alerting your healthcare provider to changes before they become emergencies. For instance, a smartwatch could alert your doctor to an irregular heartbeat, enabling immediate action.
3. **Improved Access to Care**: Telehealth bridges the gap for underserved populations, offering virtual visits to patients

in rural or remote areas, reducing travel and wait times, and even addressing mental health needs through teletherapy platforms.

THE ROLE OF TECHNOLOGY IN CARE DELIVERY

Advancements in digital health tools are enhancing patient outcomes and engagement:

- **Artificial Intelligence (AI)**: AI-driven algorithms can identify early signs of conditions like cancer or diabetic retinopathy in imaging scans. This enhances diagnostic accuracy and enables earlier interventions.
- **Robotic Surgery**: This is a rapidly growing technique. In developed countries, it is currently used in 15-20% of eligible surgeries. It is commonly used in urology (prostatectomies), gynecology (hysterectomies), and general surgery (hernia repairs and cholecystectomies).
- **Digital Therapeutics (DTx)**: Software applications designed for specific conditions, such as apps that guide patients through cognitive-behavioral therapy or digital platforms for managing asthma, are gaining traction. The DTx market is expected to grow from $3.4 billion in 2020 to $13.1 billion by 2027 (*Statista*).
- **Mobile Health Applications**: Over 350,000 health apps are now available globally, enabling users to track a wide range of health-related goals, including fitness and medication adherence. These apps provide valuable insights and reminders that help keep patients engaged in their health.

Benefits of Integration

The benefits of integration paint a future where the integration of telehealth and digital health technologies is seamless:

- **Streamlined Care**: Virtual consultations, combined with wearable data, will enable providers to view a patient's comprehensive health information without the need for in-person visits.
- **Chronic Disease Management**: Telehealth with RPM enables effective treatment of chronic conditions, such as diabetes, hypertension, and heart failure. For instance, when a continuous glucose monitor flags excessively high sugar levels in an individual patient, the telehealth visit may adjust the dosing of insulin in real time.
- **Improved Accessibility**: Virtual care, through the use of digital tools, ensures equity for patients living in rural areas or those with mobility difficulties.

Challenges to Overcome

- **Digital Divide**: Only some have reliable internet or access to devices. Bridging this gap will be critical to ensuring telehealth's inclusivity.
- **Interoperability**: Digital health platforms must integrate seamlessly with electronic health records (EHRs) to avoid fragmented care.
- **Privacy Concerns**: Strong cybersecurity measures are essential to protect sensitive health data shared during virtual visits.

INNOVATIONS IN MANAGED CARE MODELS

- **Fee-for-Service Flaws**: The traditional FFS model incentivizes high volumes of services, often resulting in unnecessary tests and treatments. This drives up costs without guaranteeing better outcomes.
- **Value-Based Care Focus**: VBC models prioritize preventive care, efficient resource use, and patient engagement. Providers are rewarded for improving health outcomes, reducing hospital readmissions, and achieving patient satisfaction.

Emerging Care Models

1. **Accountable Care Organizations (ACOs)** are groups of providers who collaborate to deliver coordinated care. They ensure patients receive the proper care at the right time and are incentivized to meet quality benchmarks and avoid unnecessary services.
2. **Patient-Centered Medical Homes (PCMHs)**: In this model, primary care teams focus on long-term relationships, addressing the whole person rather than individual conditions. This reduces hospitalizations and improves satisfaction.
3. **Population Health Management**: Using data analytics, providers target high-risk groups with preventive measures and tailored interventions, addressing medical needs and social determinants of health (SDOH).

Addressing Social Determinants of Health

Healthcare is about understanding the conditions in which people live, work, and age. Managed care organizations can help close health disparities by addressing issues related to housing, nutrition, and transportation. Programs that offer nutritious meals to diabetic patients or provide transportation to appointments for those without access to a car are examples of how addressing Social Determinants of Health (SDOH) can directly improve outcomes.

Technology-Driven Innovations

Technology is enabling more personalized, proactive care, from remote monitoring to community health workers using apps for real-time updates. For example, a remote heart failure program might use wearable devices to track vital signs, alerting providers to intervene early and prevent hospitalization.

PREPARING FOR THE FUTURE: ADAPTING TO CHANGE

The dynamic nature of healthcare requires that patients and providers be informed and adaptable. Be proactive about new technologies, care models, and insurance policies.

For Patients

- **Educate Yourself**: Understand healthcare trends and technologies through acclaimed literature.
- **Employ Technology**: Fully engage with patient portals, health apps, and wearable devices to monitor your health and facilitate communication with your providers.

- **Self-Advocate**: Have a friend or loved one advocate on your behalf. Join an advocacy group to stay up-to-date about your rights and resources.

For Providers

- **Educate Patients**: Assist patients in understanding new technologies and care models.
- **Coordinate Care**: Ensure seamless integration of digital tools and in-person visits.
- **Adapt to Policies**: Stay ahead of regulatory changes to deliver compliant, high-quality care.

THE ROAD AHEAD

Telehealth, digital health, and innovative care models continue to disrupt the healthcare sector. It has massive potential because it's personalized, accessible, efficient, equitable, and just better. Even if they get in that long line for improvement in health outcomes.

Key highlights of the future are:

- More active use of remote monitoring to manage chronic conditions more dynamically.
- More advanced value-based care models focused on prevention and coordination.
- Greater emphasis on social determinants of health, ensuring care addresses the root causes of disparities.

As healthcare continues to evolve, staying informed and engaged will empower patients and providers to achieve better outcomes and effectively navigate the complexities of managed care.

KEEPING THE GAME ALIVE

Now that you've finished this journey through The Ultimate Handbook, you have the tools to take charge of your care, advocate

Now, it's your turn to keep this knowledge alive.

By simply leaving a review on Amazon, you'll guide other readers to this life-saving resource—and share your passion for makin

Your voice matters. Your story matters. And your review could inspire others to act before it's too late.

Thank you for your support. The movement to protect patients is only alive when we pass on our stories and stand up for one an

Click here to leave your review on Amazon:

https://www.amazon.com/review/review-your-purchases/?asin=BOOKASIN

With gratitude,
Dr. Robin Snead

CONCLUSION

As we end our journey together, I want to reiterate this book's primary purpose and vision. I aim to inform you about the potential dangers of incentivizing less care within managed care systems and provide practical steps for navigating these systems to achieve better health outcomes. As an internal medicine physician with over thirty-five years of experience, I have witnessed firsthand the complexities and challenges patients face within the managed care system (MCS). This book has equipped you with the knowledge and tools to effectively advocate for yourself and your loved ones.

Throughout the chapters, we delved into various aspects of the managed care system. In **Chapter 1**, we examined the origins and evolution of managed care, focusing on the transition from fee-for-service models to managed care organizations (MCOs) and the economic and social factors that influenced this shift. We examined the structure and functioning of MCOs, including the roles of HMOs, PPOs, EPOs, and POS plans, as well as the financial mechanisms and incentives that influence provider behavior.

Chapter 2 provided a step-by-step guide to navigating the managed care system. We emphasized the importance of selecting the right plan, understanding your network, preparing for medical appointments, and keeping organized records. We also discussed strategies for overcoming common obstacles such as denied claims, referral delays, and prescription drug formularies.

Chapter 3 focused on common pitfalls within the MCS, such as long appointment wait times and prior authorization hurdles. We offered practical strategies for expediting approvals and reducing wait times, including online scheduling tools, calling during off-peak hours, and exploring alternative care options.

In **Chapter 4**, we highlighted the importance of self-advocacy in healthcare. We discussed how to educate yourself about your health conditions, build a comprehensive health history file, understand your rights as a patient, and effectively communicate with healthcare providers. We also covered navigating hospital discharges and ensuring safe transitions of care.

Chapter 5 explored the role of technology in modern healthcare, including the benefits and limitations of telehealth, electronic health records (EHRs), and health apps. We provided guidance on preparing for telehealth appointments, maximizing the use of health apps, and integrating digital tools into your healthcare routine.

In **Chapter 6**, we emphasized the importance of preventive care and wellness, discussing the benefits of preventive screenings, establishing a wellness routine, and the role of vaccinations in maintaining good health. We shared practical tips for integrating these practices into your daily life to achieve better health outcomes.

Chapter 7 addressed the challenges of managing insurance claims and out-of-pocket expenses. We provided strategies for appealing denied claims, managing healthcare expenses, and selecting the right insurance plan for your needs. We also discussed the role of health savings accounts (HSAs) and flexible spending accounts (FSAs) in managing medical costs.

In **Chapter 8**, we shared real-life case studies to illustrate the challenges and triumphs of navigating the MCS. These stories highlighted the importance of persistence, effective communication, and comprehensive documentation in securing necessary medical treatments and achieving positive health outcomes.

Chapter 9 examined the impact of COVID-19 on the healthcare system, including healthcare worker shortages, the rise of telehealth, and coping with care delays and disruptions. We provided recommendations for navigating healthcare during the pandemic, emphasizing the importance of flexibility and proactive management.

In **Chapter 10**, we discussed the growing concern of iatrogenic deaths and medical errors. We explored strategies for preventing medical errors, enhancing patient safety, and actively participating in your care to reduce the risk of adverse outcomes.

Chapter 11 focused on enhancing doctor-patient relationships, emphasizing the importance of trust, effective communication, and collaborative care. We provided practical tips for building strong relationships with your healthcare providers and ensuring comprehensive and coordinated care.

Chapter 12 addressed the challenges of navigating healthcare bureaucracy, including managing healthcare paperwork, maintaining accurate health records, and navigating the referral process. We provided strategies for organizing and managing healthcare documents, as well as ensuring effective communication between providers.

Chapter 13 highlighted the importance of addressing mental health within the MCS. We discussed recognizing and addressing mental health needs, accessing mental health services, and integrating mental and physical health care. We provided strategies for seeking mental health support and navigating insurance coverage for mental health services.

Chapter 14 focused on understanding your legal rights and patient advocacy. We discussed the fundamental rights of patients, legal recourse in cases of medical negligence, and the role of patient advocacy services. We provided practical tips for utilizing patient advocacy services and ensuring your rights are respected.

In **Chapter 15**, we explored the unique healthcare needs of special populations, including seniors, children, and individuals with chronic illnesses and disabilities. We provided strategies for navigating managed care for these populations and accessing the necessary resources and support services.

Finally, in **Chapter 16**, we looked at the future of managed care, discussing the anticipated growth of telehealth, advancements in digital health technologies, and innovations in managed care models. We emphasized the importance of staying informed, adapting to changes in healthcare, and leveraging new technologies and care models to achieve better health outcomes.

As we conclude, here are some key takeaways to remember:

1. Educate yourself about your health conditions and the managed care system.
2. Advocate for yourself and actively participate in your healthcare decisions.

3. Stay organized and keep detailed records of your medical history and treatments.
4. Build strong relationships with your healthcare providers and communicate effectively.
5. Utilize technology and digital tools to enhance your healthcare experience.
6. Stay informed about changes in healthcare and adapt to new trends and innovations.

Please take these lessons to heart and apply them in your healthcare journey. Advocate for yourself and your loved ones, stay informed, and actively engage in your care. Doing so allows you to navigate the managed care system effectively and achieve better health outcomes.

Reflecting on my journey as an internal medicine physician, I am reminded of the countless patients I have had the privilege of caring for over the years. Each patient's story is unique, but the common thread is the importance of advocacy, education, and proactive management in achieving positive health outcomes. My commitment to patient care and advocacy remains unwavering, and I hope this book has inspired you to take an active role in your healthcare.

Thank you for allowing me to share my experiences and insights with you. I wish you the best in your healthcare journey and hope that the knowledge and strategies in this book empower you to navigate the managed care system with confidence and achieve the best possible health outcomes.

ADVOCACY SERVICES

Navigating the healthcare system can be challenging, but several organizations offer patient advocacy services to help individuals manage their healthcare needs. Here are some notable patient advocate organizations and resources to help you find the support you need:

1. **Patient Advocate Foundation (PAF):** A national nonprofit organization that provides professional case management services to patients with chronic, life-threatening, and debilitating illnesses. They assist with access to care, employment maintenance, and financial stability preservation. More information is available on their website: Patient Advocate Foundation
2. **Greater National Advocates (GNA):** A nonprofit organization dedicated to raising awareness about the benefits of independent patient advocacy. GNA provides a comprehensive directory of qualified patient advocates nationwide. You can search for advocates GnaNOW

3. **National Association of Healthcare Advocacy Consultants (NAHAC):** An organization that supports the development of the health advocacy profession and provides resources for both advocates and patients. They offer a directory of healthcare advocates and consultants: Nahac
4. **Solace:** A platform that connects patients with healthcare advocates, including nurses, physician assistants, and pharmacists, to guide them through the complexities of the healthcare system. Solace's services are covered by Medicare and some Medicare Advantage : Solace Health
5. **Centers for Medicare & Medicaid Services (CMS):** CMS provides resources to help patients find advocates, including information on the Patient Advocate Foundation and guidance for veterans seeking assistance through the VA's Patient Advocacy Program: Centers for Medicare & Medicaid Services
6. **Chicago-Based Patient Advocacy Services:**
    - **Greater Chicago Advocates:** A patient advocacy network offering services in the Chicago area. Contact them at 120 W. Madison Suite 1403, Chicago, IL 60602: Chicago Advocates
    - **Chicago Patient Advocacy:** Provides professional patient healthcare advocacy services, including the development of personalized care plans: Chicago Patient Advocacy
    - **Chicago Health Advocates:** Offers personalized healthcare advocacy services, including a free thirty-minute telephone consultation to discuss how they can assist you: Chicago Health Advocates
    - **UCan Health Advocacy:** Provides empathetic support and advocacy services, connecting patients with

advocates who take on their clients' causes as their own: <u>U Can Health Advocacy</u>

When seeking a patient advocate, consider the following steps:

- **Identify Your Needs:** Determine the specific areas where you require assistance, such as understanding medical information, coordinating care, or managing insurance issues.
- **Research and Verify Credentials:** Look for advocates with relevant experience and certifications. Many organizations provide directories of qualified advocates.
- **Contact Potential Advocates:** Contact potential advocates to discuss your needs, learn about their services, and assess whether they are a good fit for you.
- **Check for Coverage:** Some advocacy services may be covered by insurance plans, including Medicare. Verify with your insurance provider to understand your options.

By utilizing these resources and taking proactive steps, you can find a patient advocate to help navigate the complexities of the healthcare system and ensure your needs are met.

I have attempted to help patients navigate through managed health care because I have seen it can be difficult over my years of practicing medicine. That being said, you must actively attempt to stay as healthy as possible.

NUTRITION TIPS

My colleague Diane Egan and I have done group medical visits in my medical office for twenty years. Diane was a naturopath and a functional nutritionist. She was brilliant and taught me a lot about her perspective on diet, nutrition, and supplements, and I integrated this into my medical practice. These are core components for good health; I will add some essential items to be considered for healthy nutrition that we consulted on in our group sessions. Mind you, these were our patients, so we knew their nutritional needs. Please talk to your doctor before adding these entries to your diet and lifestyle.

This list is pretty basic and nothing fancy, but adding these items to your diet may improve your health.

ANTI-INFLAMMATORY FOODS

1. **Fruits**:
    - Berries (blueberries, raspberries, strawberries): Rich in antioxidants and anthocyanins.

- Citrus fruits (oranges, lemons): Contain vitamin C and flavonoids.

2. **Vegetables**:
    - Leafy greens (spinach, kale, Swiss chard): Packed with vitamins A, C, and K.
    - Cruciferous vegetables (broccoli, brussels sprouts, cauliflower): Contain sulforaphane, an anti-inflammatory compound.
3. **Healthy Fats**:
    - Olive oil: High in monounsaturated fats and polyphenols.
    - Avocados: Provide anti-inflammatory compounds and fiber.
    - Fatty fish (salmon, mackerel, sardines): Rich in omega-3 fatty acids.
4. **Spices and Herbs**:
    - Turmeric (with black pepper): Contains curcumin, a powerful anti-inflammatory.
    - Ginger: Helps reduce inflammation and aids digestion.
    - Garlic: Contains allicin, which has anti-inflammatory properties.
5. **Whole Grains**:
    - Quinoa, oats, and barley: Provide fiber and reduce inflammatory markers.
6. **Nuts and Seeds**:
    - Walnuts, almonds, chia seeds, flaxseeds: Excellent sources of omega-3s and antioxidants.

NUTRIENT-PACKED FOODS

1. **Superfoods**:
   - Dark chocolate (70 percent cocoa or higher): High in flavonoids.
   - Green tea: Contains catechins, which are antioxidants.
2. **Colorful Vegetables**:
   - Sweet potatoes, carrots, and red peppers: Rich in beta-carotene.
3. **Fermented Foods**:
   - Yogurt, kefir, sauerkraut, kimchi: Support gut health with probiotics.
4. **Legumes**:
   - Lentils, chickpeas, and black beans: High in protein, fiber, and minerals.

ESSENTIAL VITAMINS AND THEIR SOURCES

1. **Vitamin D**:
   - Sources: Sunlight, fortified foods, fatty fish, egg yolks.
   - Benefits: Supports bone health, immunity, and mood regulation.
2. **Vitamin C**:
   - Sources: Citrus fruits, bell peppers, strawberries, kiwi.
   - Benefits: Boosts immune function and acts as an antioxidant.
3. **Vitamin K**:
   - Sources: Kale, spinach, and fermented soy (natto).
   - Benefits: Improves bone and cardiovascular health.
4. **Vitamin E**:
   - Sources: Almonds, sunflower seeds, spinach.
   - Benefits: Acts as an antioxidant, protecting cells.

KEY SUPPLEMENTS FOR LONGEVITY

Note: This list is not designed to be complete but a foundation on which to build.

1. **Omega-3 Fatty Acids:**
   - Sources: Fish oil or algal oil (for vegetarians).
   - Benefits: Reduces inflammation and supports heart and brain health.
2. **Magnesium:**
   - Sources: Supplements or foods like nuts, seeds, and leafy greens.
   - Benefits: Regulates muscle and nerve function and supports heart health.
3. **Probiotics:**
   - Sources: Supplement form or fermented foods.
   - Benefits: Improves gut health and reduces inflammation.
4. **Curcumin:**
   - Sources: Turmeric supplements (with piperine for better absorption).
   - Benefits: Potent anti-inflammatory and antioxidant properties.
5. **Resveratrol:**
   - Sources: Found in red wine (in moderation) or as a supplement.
   - Benefits: Antioxidant that may protect against aging-related diseases.
6. **Coenzyme Q10 (CoQ10):**
   - Benefits: Supports mitochondrial function and heart health.

7. **Multivitamins**:
   - A comprehensive multivitamin ensures all nutrient gaps are covered.

LONGEVITY STRATEGIES

1. **Intermittent Fasting**:
   - Benefits: Reduces inflammation, supports cellular repair, and improves metabolic health.
2. **Hydration**:
   - Drink plenty of water. It can be infused with lemon, cucumber, or mint for added nutrients and antioxidants.
3. **Balanced Lifestyle**:
   - Combine these foods with regular exercise, stress management, and sufficient sleep for optimal health and longevity.

EPILOGUE

As I close this book, I reflect on my journey as a physician—a path marked by dedication, resilience, and a profound sense of purpose. My parents, Bill and Queen Snead, were strong business people early in life, as my sister Joann, twenty-two years my senior, knew them well. However, my memory of them is different. My mother was plagued with a chronic debilitating illness all of my life, which gave me my unwavering desire to be a doctor.

My career began with a vision of healing, providing treatment, hope, and guidance to those in need. Over the years, I built a thriving integrative medical practice, combining traditional internal medicine with a holistic approach that embraced the whole person, not just their symptoms. I worked alongside brilliant minds like my colleague Dr. Diane Egan, a naturopath and functional nutritionist. She shared my commitment to empowering patients through education and care.

Yet, alongside this fulfilling journey, I've witnessed the harrowing transformation of healthcare into a managed system that often prioritizes cost savings over patient well-being. In its relentless quest to economize, managed healthcare has imposed bureaucratic barriers and created a culture where often doing less for patients is seen as a win. This approach has compromised the quality of care and has led to devastating mistakes—mistakes that have cost lives.

One of the most painful experiences was watching my dear friend June almost lose her life multiple times due to the system's indifference. It was only through my intervention, using my knowledge and persistence, along with her outstanding oncologist, Dr. V Amed, that we were able to navigate the maze of premature discharges and missed diagnoses to get her the care she deserved. Stories like hers are tragically not uncommon, underscoring the urgent need for change.

Through this book, I have shared anecdotal accounts of these failures—not to assign blame but to highlight the critical flaws in our system. More importantly, I have provided patients with tools and strategies to advocate for themselves. From securing prior authorizations to selecting the most effective medications and engaging advocates, these lessons are designed to empower individuals to take control of their healthcare journeys.

The reality is stark: Medical errors are the third leading cause of death in the United States, accounting for an estimated 400,000 lives lost annually. Many of these deaths are preventable. By being vigilant, informed, and proactive, patients and their loved ones can help prevent becoming part of this statistic.

As I close this chapter of my life, I remain dedicated to my mission of patient advocacy. Healthcare should be a partnership built on trust, compassion, and a shared goal of wellness. Together, we can navigate the challenges of managed care and strive for a system that values lives over ledgers.

REFERENCES

Good Monk. n.d. "40+ Health Fitness Quotes to Keep Motivated & Positive." Accessed April 7, 2025. https://www.goodmonk.in/blogs/blogs/40-health-fitness-quotes-to-keep-motivated-positive?srsltid=AfmBOopEY_bzNz2aLbb Tkiv297VrZJwQwgxgMhhxadz4L-k7fN_kibUd

"7 Steps to Improve Scheduling in Your Outpatient Practice." 2023. American Medical Association. January 19, 2023. https://www.ama-assn.org/practice-management/sustainability/7-steps-improve-scheduling-your-outpatient-practice.

Bhaumik, Kaushik, Sumitro Sarkar, and Glen Fernandes. n.d. "How Electronic Prior Authorization Can Help Health Care." EY. https://www.ey.com/en_us/insights/health/how-electronic-prior-authorization-can-help-health-care.

Bierman, Arlene S., Jing Wang, Patrick G. O'Malley, and Dina K. Moss. 2021. "Transforming Care for People with Multiple Chronic Conditions: Agency for Healthcare Research and Quality's Research Agenda." *Health Services Research* 56 (Suppl 1): 973–79. https://doi.org/10.1111/1475-6773.13863.

Bundorf, M Kate, Kevin A Schulman, Judith A Stafford, Darrell Gaskin, James G Jollis, and José J Escarce. 2004. "Impact of Managed Care on the Treatment, Costs, and Outcomes of Fee-for-Service Medicare Patients with Acute Myocardial Infarction." *Health Services Research* 39 (1): 131–52. https://doi.org/10.1111/j.1475-6773.2004.00219.x.

CDC. 2024a. "Are You Up to Date on Your Preventive Care?" Chronic Disease. November 4, 2024. https://www.cdc.gov/chronic-disease/prevention/preventive-care.html.

———. 2024b. "Child and Adolescent Immunization Schedule by Age." Vaccines & Immunizations. November 19, 2024. https://www.cdc.gov/vaccines/hcp/imz-schedules/child-adolescent-age.html.

"Checklists to Improve Patient Safety." 2025. American Hospital Association. March 11, 2025. https://www.aha.org/ahahret-guides/2013-07-10-checklists-improve-patient-safety.

"Common Reasons for a Denial and Examples of Appeal Letters." n.d. Washington State Office of the Insurance Commissioner. https://www.insurance.wa.gov/common-reasons-denial-and-examples-appeal-letters.

Definitive Healthcare. (2022). *Addressing the healthcare staffing shortage.* https://www.definitivehc.com/sites/default/files/resources/pdfs/addressing-the-healthcare-staffing-shortage-report.pdf

Džakula, Aleksandar, Danko Relić, and Paolo Michelutti. 2022. "Health Workforce Shortage – Doing the Right Things or Doing Things Right?" *Croatian Medical Journal* 63 (2): 107–9. https://doi.org/10.3325/cmj.2022.63.107.

"Effective Communication in Health Care." 2021. Tulane University. September 29, 2021. https://publichealth.tulane.edu/blog/communication-in-healthcare/.

Falkson, Samuel R., and Vijay N. Srinivasan. 2025. "Health Maintenance Organization." In *StatPearls*. Treasure Island (FL): StatPearls Publishing. http://www.ncbi.nlm.nih.gov/books/NBK554454/.

Forrest, Christopher B, Leiyu Shi, Sarah von Schrader, and Judy Ng. 2002. "Managed Care, Primary Care, and the Patient-Practitioner Relationship." *Journal of General Internal Medicine* 17 (4): 270–77. https://doi.org/10.1046/j.1525-1497.2002.10309.x.

Hale, Timothy M., and Joseph C. Kvedar. 2014. "Privacy and Security Concerns in Telehealth." *AMA Journal of Ethics* 16 (12): 981–85. https://doi.org/10.1001/virtualmentor.2014.16.12.jdsc1-1412.

Haque, Mainul, Judy McKimm, Massimo Sartelli, Sameer Dhingra, Francesco M Labricciosa, Salequl Islam, Dilshad Jahan, et al. 2020. "Strategies to Prevent Healthcare-Associated Infections: A Narrative Overview." *Risk Management and Healthcare Policy* 13 (September):1765–80. https://doi.org/10.2147/RMHP.S269315.

"HMO vs PPO: Differences, Similarities & Things to Consider." n.d. CareFirst BlueCross BlueShield. https://individual.carefirst.com/individuals-families/health-insurance-basics/how-health-insurance-works/hmo-vs-ppo.page.

"Home." 2024. Patient Advocate Foundation. May 14, 2024. https://www.patientadvocate.org/.

Houlihan, Bethlyn, Miriam Brody, Andrea Plant, Sarah Everhart Skeels, Judi Zazula, Diana Pernigotti, Christa Green, Stathis Hasiotis, and Alan Jette. 2016. "Health Care Self-Advocacy Strategies for Negotiating Health Care Environments: Analysis of Recommendations by Satisfied Consumers with SCI and SCI Practitioners." *Topics in Spinal Cord Injury Rehabilitation* 22 (1): 13–26. https://doi.org/10.1310/sci2201-13.

"How to Appeal an Insurance Company Decision." n.d. HealthCare.Gov. https://www.healthcare.gov/appeal-insurance-company-decision/.

"How to Speed up Your Prior Authorization Process Using Electronic Health Records Data Exchange." 2024. American Medical Association. May 3, 2024. https://www.ama-assn.org/practice-management/prior-authorization/how-speed-your-prior-authorization-process-using-electronic.

"Impact of the COVID-19 Pandemic on the Hospital and Outpatient Clinician Workforce: Challenges and Policy Responses." 2022. ASPE. May 3, 2022. http://aspe.hhs.gov/reports/covid-19-health-care-workforce.

Jalali, Faride Sadat, Parisa Bikineh, and Sajad Delavari. 2021. "Strategies for Reducing out of Pocket Payments in the Health System: A Scoping Review." *Cost Effectiveness and Resource Allocation: C/E* 19 (August):47. https://doi.org/10.1186/s12962-021-00301-8.

Johns Hopkins Medicine. (n.d.). *Study suggests medical errors now third leading cause of death in the U.S.* https://www.hopkinsmedicine.org/news/media/releases/study_suggests_medical_errors_now_third_leading_cause_of_death_in_the_us

Liang, Katherine, and Eric Alper. 2018. "Patient Safety During Hospital Discharge." *Patient Safety During Hospital Discharge*, April. https://psnet.ahrq.gov/perspective/patient-safety-during-hospital-discharge.

"Managed Care." 2025. In *Wikipedia*. https://en.wikipedia.org/w/index.php?title=Managed_care&oldid=1275728707.

Makary, M. A., & Daniel, M. (2016). Medical error—the third leading cause of death in the US. *BMJ*, 353, i2139. https://doi.org/10.1136/bmj.i2139

Meryn, Siegfried. 1998. "Improving Doctor-Patient Communication." *BMJ : British Medical Journal* 316 (7149): 1922–30. https://www.ncbi.nlm.nih.gov/pmc/articles/PMC1113402/.

"Mobile Apps for Chronic Diseases Management | Top Chronic Illness Apps." 2022. *DelveInsight Business Research* (blog). May 11, 2022. https://www.delveinsight.com/blog/chronic-disease-management-apps.

Monaghesh, Elham, and Alireza Hajizadeh. 2020. "The Role of Telehealth during COVID-19 Outbreak: A Systematic Review Based on Current Evidence." *BMC Public Health* 20 (August):1193. https://doi.org/10.1186/s12889-020-09301-4.

Moradell, Ana, José Antonio Casajús, Luis A. Moreno, Germán Vicente-Rodríguez, and Alba Gómez-Cabello. 2023. "Effects of Diet—Exercise Interaction on Human Health across a Lifespan." *Nutrients* 15 (11): 2520. https://doi.org/10.3390/nu15112520.

Parsi, Kayhan. 2001. "Financial Incentives in Managed Care." *AMA Journal of Ethics* 3 (1): 3. https://doi.org/10.1001/virtualmentor.2001.3.1.hlaw1-0101.

"Patients' Bill of Rights." n.d. U.S. Office of Personnel Management. Accessed March 12, 2025. https://www.opm.gov/healthcare-insurance/healthcare/reference-materials/bill-of-rights/.

Pearson, Steven D, and Lisa H Raeke. 2000. "Patients' Trust in Physicians: Many Theories, Few Measures, and Little Data." *Journal of General Internal Medicine* 15 (7): 509–13. https://doi.org/10.1046/j.1525-1497.2000.11002.x.

Rodziewicz, Thomas L., Benjamin Houseman, Sarosh Vaqar, and John E. Hipskind.

2025. "Medical Error Reduction and Prevention." In *StatPearls*. Treasure Island (FL): StatPearls Publishing. http://www.ncbi.nlm.nih.gov/books/NBK499956/.

Safety, Institute of Medicine (US) Committee on Optimizing Graduate Medical Trainee (Resident) Hours and Work Schedule to Improve Patient, Cheryl Ulmer, Dianne Miller Wolman, and Michael M. E. Johns. 2009. "System Strategies to Improve Patient Safety and Error Prevention." In *Resident Duty Hours: Enhancing Sleep, Supervision, and Safety*. National Academies Press (US). https://www.ncbi.nlm.nih.gov/books/NBK214937/.

Stelter, Nicole. 2023. "Collaborative Care: An Integrated Care Model That Works." Blue Shield of California News Center. November 8, 2023. https://news.blueshieldca.com/2023/11/08/collaborative-care-an-integrated-care-model-that-works.

"Steps to Appeal a Health Insurance Claim Denial." n.d. CareFirst BlueCross BlueShield. https://individual.carefirst.com/individuals-families/health-insurance-basics/health-insurance-costs/steps-to-appeal-claim-denial.page.

"Telehealth in the Pandemic—How Has It Changed Health Care Delivery in Medicaid and Medicare?" 2025. U.S. GAO. January 7, 2025. https://www.gao.gov/blog/telehealth-pandemic-how-has-it-changed-health-care-delivery-medicaid-and-medicare.

"The Managed Care Answer Guide." n.d. Patient Advocate Foundation. https://www.patientadvocate.org/wp-content/uploads/Managed-Care-Answer-Guide.pdf.

"The Simple Guide to Health Plans." n.d. Aetna. Accessed March 12, 2025. https://www.aetna.com/health-guide/hmo-pos-ppo-hdhp-whats-the-difference.html.

Upadhyay, Soumya, and Han-fen Hu. 2022. "A Qualitative Analysis of the Impact of Electronic Health Records (EHR) on Healthcare Quality and Safety: Clinicians' Lived Experiences." *Health Services Insights* 15 (March):11786329211070722. https://doi.org/10.1177/11786329211070722.

Yarnall, K. S. H., Pollak, K. I., Østbye, T., Krause, K. M., & Michener, J. L. (2003). Primary care: Is there enough time for prevention? *American Journal of Public Health*, 93(4), 635–641. https://doi.org/10.2105/AJPH.93.4.635

Vogel, Susanna. 2023. "Healthcare Worker Exodus Continued through 2022, New Data Shows." Healthcare Dive. October 17, 2023. https://www.healthcaredive.com/news/healthcare-worker-exodus-physician-burnout-definitive/696769/.

Wallack, Stanley S. 1992. "Managed Care: Practice, Pitfalls, and Potential." *Health Care Financing Review* 1991 (Suppl): 27–34. https://www.ncbi.nlm.nih.gov/pmc/articles/PMC4195142/.

Wang, Ming-Jye, and Yi-Ting Lo. 2022. "Strategies for Improving the Utilization of Preventive Care Services: Application of Importance–Performance Gap

Analysis Method." *International Journal of Environmental Research and Public Health* 19 (20): 13195. https://doi.org/10.3390/ijerph192013195.

AUTHOR'S BIO

Dr. Robin Snead, MD, is a dedicated physician and an unwavering advocate for patient care whose career spans over 35 years of transformative work in internal medicine and integrative healthcare. A Northwestern University School of Medicine graduate, Dr. Snead honed her expertise during her residency at Rush Presbyterian St. Luke's Hospital, laying a strong foundation for her mission to provide compassionate, patient-centered care.

Throughout her career, Dr. Snead has been a trailblazer, pioneering a progressive integrative medical practice that combined traditional medicine with holistic approaches. For over two decades in her medical office, she helped lead group sessions alongside a Naprapath and functional nutritionist, Dr. Diane Egan, educating patients on managing chronic conditions such as diabetes, hypertension, and cardiovascular disease. Her practice not only healed but empowered, emphasizing education, lifestyle changes, and preventive measures.

Dr. Snead's dedication extended beyond her practice. She trained future healthcare providers, and contributed to the evolution of healthcare systems through her roles as a managing partner of the Doctor's Office Center. Her commitment to improving patient outcomes has been recognized in groundbreaking initiatives such as Physician Quality Care, where, as a founding board member, she helped establish one of the early physician-owned IPAs, in the 1990's featured in *Chicago Magazine*.

Dr. Snead owned WSW a company where she employed LCSWs and went out and performed group mental health therapy on elderly and disabled patients in nursing homes.

Despite her accomplishments, Dr. Snead has witnessed the dark side of managed healthcare, which often prioritizes cost-cutting over patient safety and well-being. These experiences have fueled her passion for advocacy and inspired her to write this book. Through compelling anecdotes and actionable strategies, she equips readers with the tools to navigate the healthcare system, avoid medical errors, and advocate effectively for their care.

Dr. Snead has two adult children, Lawrence and Sade Larkin. A daughter-in-law, Blessing Larkin, and a rambunctious grandson, Zion. She works in telemedicine seeing mental health patients, leveraging her expertise to reach diverse patient populations. Her story is a testament to resilience, innovation, and a commitment to the art of healing.

www.ingramcontent.com/pod-product-compliance
Lightning Source LLC
Chambersburg PA
CBHW060823050426
42453CB00008B/571